PRIMARY PRACTICE PAPERS

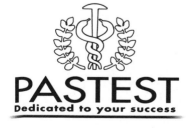

PASTEST
Dedicated to your success

Dedicated to my wife, Kate, for her patience and understanding, and our boys Alex and Dominic.

FRCA PRIMARY PRACTICE PAPERS

Tim Isitt MRCP FRCA
Consultant Anaesthetist,
Luton and Dunstable Hospital NHS Trust
London

© 2000 PASTEST
Egerton Court
Parkgate Estate
Knutsford
Cheshire WA16 8DX

Telephone: 01565 752000

First edition 2000
Reprinted 2005

ISBN: 1 901198 39 1

A catalogue record for this book is available from the British Library.

The information contained within this book was obtained by the authors from reliable sources. However, while every effort has been made to ensure its accuracy, no responsibility for loss, damage or injury occasioned to any person acting or refraining from action as a result of information contained herein can be accepted by the publishers or authors.

Typeset by Breeze Limited, Manchester.
Printed and bound by Hobbs the Printers Ltd, Totton, Hampshire.

CONTENTS

CONTRIBUTORS

Anne Campbell FRCA
Specialist Registrar in Anaesthetics
The Middlesex Hospital
London

Sarah Chieveley-Williams MBBS(Hons) MRCP FRCA
Clinical Research Fellow
The Middlesex Hospital
London

Ailsa Evans MBChB FRCA
Consultant Anaesthetist
Royal National Throat, Nose and Ear Hospital
London

INTRODUCTION

In 1996 the FRCA Diploma was restructured from a three to a two part examination – the Primary and the Final.

To take the Primary exam a trainee must have completed a minimum of 12 months of recognised training, although it is generally accepted that most trainees will not attempt the exam until they have completed 18 months training.

Candidates are allowed a maximum of four attempts at the exam, and are referred for advice and counselling after two failures.

THE EXAMINATION

The examination is divided into two parts:

1. The Multiple Choice Questions Paper (MCQs)

90 questions, each with 5 stems, are to be completed in 3 hours
These questions consist of:
30 in Physiology and Biochemistry
30 in Pharmacology
30 in Physics and Clinical Measurement

2. The Objective Structured Clinical Examination (OSCE)

16 stations to be completed in 2 hours

3. Viva 1

15 minutes Pharmacology and Statistics
15 minutes Physiology and Biochemistry

4. Viva 2

15 minutes Physics, Safety and Clinical measurement
15 minutes Clinical topics (including critical incidents)

The MCQ paper is negatively marked. Thus for each of the questions it is possible to score +1 for a correct answer, −1 for a wrong answer and 0 for an answer left blank or don't know. A total score for all 90 questions with 5 branches for each question, is then counted up.
This score will be somewhere between −450 and +450, hopefully nearer to the latter!

Candidates will then be assigned an overall grade 1, 1+, 2 or 2+. A score of 1 is an absolute fail. A score of 1+ is a borderline fail and to pass the overall examination after a 1+ score the candidate must then get a 2 or a 2+ in all the other parts of the examination in order to pass the Primary. A score of 2 is a pass and 2+ is a good pass.

A score of 1 in any part of the exam, no matter how good the other scores are, is an automatic overall fail.

The MCQ paper is traditionally felt to be the most difficult part of the exam. In one of the 1996 sittings only 30.5% of candidates passed the MCQ paper.

There is always much debate about the best way to answer MCQs and in the end it has to be up to the individual to find the technique that suits him or her best.

For some people educated guesses seem to be worth trying whilst others find that they invariably guess wrongly. The big hazard with guessing, especially if you fall into the category of bad guessers, is that the paper is negatively marked.

It is probably worth practising guessing before the real exam to try to establish whether you are a good or a bad guesser.

The MCQs in this book are accompanied by explanations to the answers, so that they are designed primarily to be educational.

There are two ways of working through this book. One way is to do the three papers under strict, timed conditions to simulate the exam and then see how you score at the end. The other, which may be more useful if you are some time away from taking the exam, is to work through the MCQs one by one.

Having answered a question, one can then read the topic in greater depth in the journals or a standard textbook. That should both consolidate existing knowledge and hopefully add further knowledge. Thus when a similar question is encountered in the future, a better score should be obtained.

The only way to really prepare for the MCQ paper is by doing a large number of MCQs and finding the technique that suits you best.

Good luck!

Tim Isitt

ABBREVIATIONS

ACTH	Adrenocorticotrophic hormone
ADH	Anti-diuretic hormone
AMP	Adenosine monophosphate
APTT	Activated partial thromboplastin time
ARDS	Acute respiratory distress syndrome
AST	Aspartate aminotransferase
a-vO$_2$	Arteriovenous oxygen gradient
BE	Base excess
BMR	Basal metabolic rate
CI	Cardiac Index
Cl	Clearance
CO	Cardiac output
CSF	Cerebrospinal fluid
CVP	Central venous pressure
DPPC	Dipalmitoyl phosphatidyl choline
FFA	Free fatty acid
FFP	Fresh frozen plasma
FGF	Fresh gas flow
FRC	Functional residual capacity
GABA	Gamma aminobutyric acid
GFR	Glomerular filtration rate
HbA	Haemoglobin A
HbF	Haemoglobin F
HME	Heat and moisture exchanger
IABP	Intra-aortic balloon pump
IBP	Invasive blood pressure
INR	International normalised ratio
IPPV	Intermittent positive pressure ventilation
LMA	Laryngeal mask airway
LOS	Lower oesophageal sphincter
MAC	Minimum alveolar concentration
mRNA	Messenger ribonucleic acid

N$_2$O	Nitrous oxide
NMDA	N-methyl-D-aspartate
PAH	Para amino hippuric acid
PT	Prothrombin time
SNP	Sodium nitroprusside
STP	Standard temperature and pressure
SV	Stroke volume
SVP	Saturated vapour pressure
SVRI	Systemic vascular resistance index
TEG	Thromboelastograph
TENS	Transcutaneous electrical nerve stimulation
TOE	Transoesophageal echo
TPN	Total parenteral nutrition
TPR	Total peripheral resistance
Vd	Volume of distribution
VIC	Vaporiser inside a circle
VOC	Vaporiser outside a circle

RECOMMENDED READING LIST

There are many excellent textbooks on the market. Listed below are the books I found personally of great use for the Primary FRCA examination.

Anatomy for Anaethetists: Ellis H and Feldman S, 7th edition, Blackwell Science Ltd.

Review of Medical Physiology: Ganong W F, 18th edition, Lange Medical Publishers.

Basic Physics and Measurement in Anaesthesia: Parbrook G D, 4th edition, Butterworth Heinemann.

Pharmacology for Anaesthetists: Calvey T N, 2nd edition, Blackwell Science Ltd.

Respiratory Physiology: West J B, 6th edition, Lippincott, Williams and Wilkins.

Lecture Notes on Clinical Medicine: Rubenstein D, 5th edition, Blackwell Science Ltd.

A-Z of Anaesthesia: Yentis S, Hirsch N P and Smith G P, 2nd edition, Butterworth Heinemann.

Clinical Textbook of Anaesthesia: Aitkinhead A R and Jones R M, Churchill Livingstone.

Acute Medicine Algorithm: Singer M and Webb A, Oxford University Press.

Essays and MCQs in Anaesthesia and Intensive Care: Murphy P M, Edward Arnold.

Handbook of Clinical Anaesthesia: Goldstone J C and Pollard B J, Churchill Livingstone.

Intensive Care: Hinds C J, 2nd edition, Ballière Tindall.

Key Topics in Anaesthesia: Craft T and Upton P, 2nd edition, Bios.

PRACTICE EXAMINATION 1

MULTIPLE CHOICE QUESTION PAPER 1

90 Questions: time allowed 3 hours.
Indicate your answers with a tick or cross in the spaces provided.

1.1   Dopamine antagonists

❑   A   increase gastric emptying
❑   B   cause tachyarrhythmias
❑   C   cause extrapyramidal effects
❑   D   cause renal artery dilation
❑   E   are anti-emetic

1.2   Diamorphine

❑   A   is less potent than morphine
❑   B   is not used in terminal illness because it is addictive
❑   C   is more rapid in action than morphine
❑   D   is more euphoric than morphine
❑   E   has a high first pass metabolism

1.3   Alfentanil

❑   A   is more potent than fentanyl
❑   B   is more lipid soluble than fentanyl
❑   C   causes myocardial depression
❑   D   may cause muscle rigidity
❑   E   is more rapid in action than fentanyl

1.4   Methohexitone

❑   A   is a thiobarbiturate
❑   B   is contraindicated in acute intermittent porphyria
❑   C   is less potent than thiopentone
❑   D   is protein bound
❑   E   is excreted unchanged in the urine

1.5 Propofol

- ❑ A is presented in 10% soya bean oil
- ❑ B decreases blood pressure mainly by vasodilatation
- ❑ C is broken down by plasma cholinesterase
- ❑ D 4–5 mg/kg is the standard induction dose in healthy adults
- ❑ E is more respiratory depressant than thiopentone

1.6 Regarding non-depolarising neuromuscular block

- ❑ A fasciculations occur prior to blockade
- ❑ B neostigmine acts by inhibiting the breakdown of acetyl choline
- ❑ C partial block is indicated by post-tetanic facilitation
- ❑ D metabolic acidosis causes prolongation
- ❑ E aminoglycoside antibiotics cause prolongation

1.7 Atracurium

- ❑ A is metabolised by ester hydrolysis
- ❑ B metabolism is slowed by hypothermia
- ❑ C breakdown produces laudanosine
- ❑ D in larger doses, is faster in onset than suxamethonium
- ❑ E a decrease in pH will increase its shelf life

1.8 Positive inotropic agents include

- ❑ A glucagon
- ❑ B potassium
- ❑ C verapamil
- ❑ D propranolol
- ❑ E theophylline

1.9　The following are metabolised in the liver:

- ❑　A　morphine
- ❑　B　atracurium
- ❑　C　procaine
- ❑　D　thiopentone
- ❑　E　vecuronium

1.10　Bupivacaine

- ❑　A　is more potent than lignocaine
- ❑　B　has a longer duration of action than lignocaine
- ❑　C　is contraindicated in intravenous regional anaesthesia
- ❑　D　is highly protein bound
- ❑　E　cardiotoxicity is associated with the D stereoisomer

1.11　Enzyme induction occurs with

- ❑　A　phenytoin
- ❑　B　phenobarbitone
- ❑　C　cimetidine
- ❑　D　carbamazepine
- ❑　E　metronidazole

1.12　Cytochrome P450 is

- ❑　A　found in lysosomes
- ❑　B　found in hepatocytes
- ❑　C　found in the endoplasmic recticulum
- ❑　D　found in the mitochondria
- ❑　E　responsible for the oxidation and reduction of drugs

1.13   pH alters the structure of

☐   A   atracurium
☐   B   midazolam
☐   C   diazepam
☐   D   suxamethonium
☐   E   morphine

1.14   Metoclopramide causes

☐   A   increased prolactin secretion
☐   B   hypertension
☐   C   oculogyric crisis
☐   D   increased lower oesophageal tone
☐   E   nausea

1.15   Reduction in uterine tone is caused by

☐   A   halothane
☐   B   amyl nitrate
☐   C   beta adrenoreceptor agonists
☐   D   neostigmine
☐   E   labetalol

1.16   Rate of transfer across the placenta depends upon

☐   A   the size of the molecule
☐   B   the lipid solubility of the molecule
☐   C   the blood flow to the placenta
☐   D   the duration of the pregnancy
☐   E   the fetal haemoglobin

1.17 **The following cause a reduction in the cerebrovascular resistance:**

❑ A enflurane
❑ B thiopentone
❑ C ether
❑ D isoflurane
❑ E fentanyl

1.18 **The following contaminants of nitrous oxide cause pulmonary oedema:**

❑ A nitric oxide
❑ B nitrogen dioxide
❑ C ammonia
❑ D carbon monoxide
❑ E nitrogen

1.19 **Nifedipine**

❑ A causes tremor
❑ B causes increased cardiac output
❑ C causes vasodilatation
❑ D is not absorbed orally
❑ E is synergistic in its action with halothane

1.20 **Ropivacaine**

❑ A is a racemic mixture
❑ B is less cardiotoxic than bupivacaine
❑ C is more potent than bupivacaine
❑ D has the same pKa as bupivacaine
❑ E produces greater motor block than bupivacaine

1.21   With regard to magnesium

☐   A   it is an anticonvulsant
☐   B   it is a neuromuscular blocking drug
☐   C   it causes cardiac arrhythmias
☐   D   the normal plasma level is 1 mmol/l
☐   E   the plasma level is controlled by calcitonin

1.22   Isoflurane

☐   A   reduces systemic vascular resistance
☐   B   reduces cardiac output
☐   C   reduces stroke volume
☐   D   causes a dose dependent drop in blood pressure
☐   E   increases heart rate

1.23   Propofol

☐   A   is dissolved in propylene glycol
☐   B   is metabolised in the liver
☐   C   causes less respiratory depression than thiopentone
☐   D   reduces the blood pressure
☐   E   has a pH of 7

1.24   The following have anticonvulsant activity:

☐   A   clonazepam
☐   B   thiopentone
☐   C   ethosuximide
☐   D   ketamine
☐   E   chlormethiazole

1.25   Suxamethonium

- ❑ A   causes a decrease in heart rate in repeated doses
- ❑ B   competes with procaine for acetylcholinesterase
- ❑ C   prolongs subsequent block with atracurium
- ❑ D   is effective and painless by the i.m. route
- ❑ E   is stable in solution

1.26   Vecuronium

- ❑ A   is a monoquaternary amine
- ❑ B   inhibits noradrenaline re-uptake at clinical doses
- ❑ C   provides as effective a block as suxamethonium at 60 seconds
- ❑ D   has a dose dependent duration of action
- ❑ E   is dependent on renal excretion

1.27   Ketamine

- ❑ A   reduces bronchial secretions
- ❑ B   is dangerous in patients with angina
- ❑ C   is dangerous in patients with asthma
- ❑ D   is stable in solution
- ❑ E   is excreted unchanged in the urine

1.28   Atenolol is

- ❑ A   a non-selective beta antagonist
- ❑ B   safe in asthmatics
- ❑ C   safe in renal failure
- ❑ D   safe in diabetics
- ❑ E   a negative inotrope

1.29   The half-life of lignocaine is increased by

- ❏ A   increasing age
- ❏ B   plasma acetylcholinesterase
- ❏ C   propranolol
- ❏ D   phenobarbitone
- ❏ E   haemorrhagic shock

1.30   Amiodarone

- ❏ A   is a hydroxy quinolone compound
- ❏ B   can cause hypoparathyroidism in long-term administration
- ❏ C   is associated with corneal deposits
- ❏ D   is used to treat supraventricular tachycardia in the presence of adrenergic blockade
- ❏ E   has a half-life of 9 hours

1.31   The following electrolyte changes occur:

- ❏ A   hypocalcaemia with hyperparathyroidism
- ❏ B   hypercalcaemia with acute pancreatitis
- ❏ C   hypoglycaemia with phaeochromocytoma
- ❏ D   hyperkalaemia with malignant hyperpyrexia
- ❏ E   hyponatraemia with TURP syndrome

1.32   Physiological changes in pregnancy include

- ❏ A   an increase in functional residual capacity
- ❏ B   the oxyhaemoglobin dissociation curve is shifted to the left
- ❏ C   anaemia, which is usually due to a fall in red cell mass
- ❏ D   increased lower oesophageal sphincter tone
- ❏ E   an increase in systemic vascular resistance

1.33 Regarding bleeding disorders

☐ A bleeding is likely when the platelet count reaches a level of $140 \times 10^9/l$

☐ B bleeding time is increased in haemophilia

☐ C excessive bleeding following multiple transfusions with stored blood or large volumes of crystalloid, is mainly due to deficiency of platelets and factors V and VIII

☐ D all coagulation proteins are synthesised by the liver and require vitamin K for their synthesis

☐ E bleeding due to excessive warfarin is rapidly corrected by vitamin K

1.34 Regarding deep vein thrombosis (DVT)

☐ A the incidence of DVT has not fallen despite the use of prophylactic anti-thrombotic measures

☐ B the treatment of small post-operative pulmonary embolism is thrombolytic therapy (e.g. streptokinase)

☐ C the risk of DVT is higher with knee and hip operations than with other surgical procedures

☐ D epidurals and spinals are absolutely contraindicated in patients receiving prophylactic subcutaneous heparin

☐ E it is advisable to discontinue HRT in women undergoing an elective surgical procedure

1.35 A 30-year-old man has the following blood gas analysis breathing air: pH 7.54, PaO_2 55 mmHg (7.2 kPa), $PaCO_2$ 25 mmHg (3.3 kPa). The following conditions could account for such results:

☐ A carbon monoxide poisoning

☐ B ascent to high altitude

☐ C spontaneous pneumothorax

☐ D hysteria

☐ E salicylate poisoning

1.36 Acute hypovolaemia leads to the following physiological changes:

- ❑ A   increased physiological dead space
- ❑ B   hypoxaemia
- ❑ C   raised arterial $PaCO_2$
- ❑ D   increased renal blood flow
- ❑ E   increased alveolar to arterial oxygen gradient

1.37 A bleeding disorder in which there is no clot retraction could be due to deficiency of

- ❑ A   platelets
- ❑ B   prothrombin
- ❑ C   calcium ions
- ❑ D   fibrinogen
- ❑ E   vitamin K

1.38 An increased arterial $PaCO_2$ is associated with

- ❑ A   increased adrenaline release
- ❑ B   tachycardia
- ❑ C   hypertension
- ❑ D   increased catecholamine release
- ❑ E   increased sweating

1.39 A Valsalva manoeuvre

- ❑ A   is a forced expiration against a closed glottis or other airway obstruction
- ❑ B   is initially associated with increased systolic arterial pressure
- ❑ C   is associated with decreased peripheral resistance
- ❑ D   is normally associated with a tachycardia
- ❑ E   is normally associated with a bradycardia

1.40 Albumin

- ❏ A has a molecular weight of approximately 65,000 Daltons
- ❏ B is increased in liver disease
- ❏ C is increased in malabsorption syndrome
- ❏ D makes a significant contribution to plasma oncotic pressure
- ❏ E has a normal value of 34–45 g/l

1.41 The minute volume is

- ❏ A reduced during sleep
- ❏ B reduced by a rise in body temperature
- ❏ C reduced by an increase in body acidity
- ❏ D increased in hypothermia
- ❏ E increased by arrival at an altitude of 5,000 m

1.42 The haemoglobin-oxygen dissociation curve is moved to the right by

- ❏ A acidosis
- ❏ B raised body temperature
- ❏ C an increase in body acidity
- ❏ D ageing
- ❏ E anaemia

1.43 In the normal heart

- ❏ A blood in the left atrium contains less oxygen than the blood in the pulmonary artery
- ❏ B right ventricular pressure might be 25/10 mmHg
- ❏ C pulmonary artery systolic pressure is usually about 10 mmHg less than right ventricular systolic pressure
- ❏ D left ventricular pressure might be 125/3 mmHg
- ❏ E blood in the pulmonary artery has an oxygen saturation of 75%

1.44   Transmitters at the autonomic ganglia include

☐ A   5HT
☐ B   glycine
☐ C   acetylcholine
☐ D   butylcholine
☐ E   noradrenaline

1.45   Reabsorption of sodium in the kidney

☐ A   is regulated by ADH
☐ B   occurs in the proximal tubule
☐ C   occurs by active transport in the loop of Henle
☐ D   is influenced by Starling's forces
☐ E   is associated with chloride reabsorption

1.46   Block of the cervical sympathetic ganglia causes

☐ A   dilatation of the conjunctival vessels
☐ B   anhidrosis of the ipsilateral face
☐ C   miosis
☐ D   nasal congestion
☐ E   enophthalmos

1.47   Metabolic acidosis can be caused by

☐ A   a pancreatic fistula
☐ B   hypoventilation
☐ C   severe diarrhoea
☐ D   renal failure
☐ E   transplantation of the ureters into the colon

1.48 **Results of prolonged severe vomiting, complicating pyloric stenosis include**

❑ A hyperchloraemia
❑ B impaired renal bicarbonate excretion
❑ C hyperventilation
❑ D acidic urine excretion
❑ E hypokalaemia

1.49 **ABO blood groups**

❑ A are an example of Mendelian dominant inheritance
❑ B may be detected in saliva
❑ C are independent of Rhesus blood groups
❑ D AB blood can be given to A and B recipients
❑ E O negative blood can be given to anyone

1.50 **The following are likely to occur in the first 10 minutes of accidental insertion of the endotracheal tube into the right main bronchus:**

❑ A arterial hypotension
❑ B severe hypercapnia
❑ C apparent increase in inhalation anaesthetic requirement
❑ D increased inflation pressure
❑ E collapse of the right upper lobe

1.51 **The normal arterial pH**

❑ A has a hydrogen ion concentration of 40 mmol/litre
❑ B is maintained by excreting approximately 60 mmol of hydrogen ions per day
❑ C is calculated from the measured pCO_2 and bicarbonate in blood gas analysers
❑ D is maintained principally by intracellular buffering systems
❑ E is slightly higher in the neonate than in the adult

1.52   In the normal ECG

❏   A   the PR interval is the total time for actual polarisation
❏   B   the QT interval measures less than 0.44 second
❏   C   the normal PR interval is 0.06–1 second
❏   D   a QRS complex duration greater than 0.1 second equals a conduction delay
❏   E   the ST interval is the time for ventricular repolarisation

1.53   When calculating lung volumes

❏   A   the anatomical dead space may be estimated using the Bohr equation
❏   B   the Vd/Vt is normally 0.3 at rest
❏   C   the FRC cannot be measured directly
❏   D   changes in expired nitrogen concentration may be used to determine closing volume
❏   E   changes in expired nitrogen concentration may be used to determine residual volume

1.54   When measuring glomerular filtration rate (GFR)

❏   A   renal blood flow must be measured or estimated
❏   B   the indicator substance used must not undergo reabsorption following tubular excretion
❏   C   the result matches the clearance of the indicator if it is really inert
❏   D   using sodium as an indicator gives an erroneously high GFR
❏   E   the average value for an adult male would be 125 ml/min

1.55   With regard to basal metabolic rate (BMR)

❏   A   BMR is the energy output of the individual at rest at room temperature
❏   B   for every 1 degree centigrade rise in body temperature, the BMR increases by 8%
❏   C   carbohydrates stimulate BMR more than proteins
❏   D   BMR increases with age
❏   E   BMR is higher in males than in females

1.56   Regarding total parenteral nutrition (TPN)

❏   A   the entire calorific requirement can be provided by glucose
❏   B   daily nitrogen requirements are greater in the elderly than in the young patient
❏   C   amino acids are provided as dextro isomers
❏   D   the use of enteral feeding is associated with a lower infection rate
❏   E   glutamine is available in most commercial amino acid preparations

1.57   The measurement of cardiac output by thermodilution

❏   A   is accurate and easily repeatable
❏   B   involves measuring the integral of temperature change over time
❏   C   the latent heat of vaporisation is used in the calculations
❏   D   is also known as the Fick technique
❏   E   may be inaccurate due to respiratory changes in the pulmonary artery temperature

1.58   The Glasgow Coma Scale

❑   A   acts as a guide to the severity of a head injury
❑   B   is a prognostic guide
❑   C   score of 2 is incompatible with survival
❑   D   gives a score of 3 if the patient's best motor response to pain is flexion
❑   E   is useless in paediatric patients

1.59   When measuring central venous pressure (CVP)

❑   A   +5 mmHg is higher than +5 mmH$_2$O
❑   B   CVP is a reliable indicator of left ventricular function
❑   C   the catheter should be in the right atrium
❑   D   a normal CVP excludes the diagnosis of pulmonary oedema
❑   E   the value of the CVP measurement is unaffected by therapeutic vasoconstriction

1.60   Pulse oximetry

❑   A   gives a falsely low reading in the presence of tricuspid incompetence
❑   B   is designed to measure light absorption every 0.5 seconds
❑   C   gives a rapid response to changes in alveolar gas tensions
❑   D   the light measurement comes from a filtered light source
❑   E   can give a falsely high reading in heavy smokers due to the carboxyhaemoglobin concentration

1.61   In an explosion

❑   A   the speed of reaction is greatest with a stoichiometric concentration
❑   B   the reaction is more vigorous with oxygen than with nitrous oxide
❑   C   1 microjoule of energy is sufficient for reactions in oxygen
❑   D   the likelihood of sparking is reduced by keeping the relative humidity greater than 50% and the temperature more than 20°C
❑   E   the stoichiometric concentration of a fuel and oxidising agent is the concentration at which an explosion occurs

1.62   When assessing neuromuscular blockade

❑ A   double burst stimulation is of particular value when there is no
          train of four present
❑ B   double burst stimulation is two short tetanic stimuli 750
          milliseconds apart
❑ C   train of four stimulation consists of 4 pulses at 2 Hz
❑ D   a fading pattern of train of four excludes prolongation of
          suxamethonium
❑ E   use of facial nerve over-estimates the degree of neuromuscular
          blockade

1.63   With regard to diathermy

❑ A   it uses an alternating current of 0.5–1 mHz
❑ B   a sine wave pattern is used for cutting
❑ C   it can act as an ignition source for bowel gas
❑ D   bipolar diathermy requires the use of a diathermy plate
❑ E   bipolar diathermy is safer in patients with pacemakers

1.64   Measures taken to minimise heat loss during surgery include

❑ A   operating theatre temperature at 20°C
❑ B   giving fluids into central vein
❑ C   humidifying inspired gases
❑ D   small doses of phenothiazines
❑ E   the use of space blankets

**1.65   The following may lead to the over-estimation of blood
            pressure:**

❑ A   using too wide a cuff
❑ B   a fat arm in a standard cuff
❑ C   letting the cuff down too slowly
❑ D   having the sphygmomanometer above the patient
❑ E   severe atherosclerosis

1.66   The saturated vapour pressure of a liquid

❏ A   is linearly related to temperature
❏ B   can exceed the normal atmospheric pressure
❏ C   is a function of barometric pressure
❏ D   is 32 kPa for isoflurane at 20°C
❏ E   is 7.6 kPa for water at 37°C

1.67   For laminar flow in a tube, the flow rate is directly proportional to

❏ A   its length
❏ B   the fourth power of its radius
❏ C   the density of the gas or liquid flowing through it
❏ D   the pressure drop across it
❏ E   the viscosity of the gas or liquid flowing across it

1.68   Helium has the following advantages over nitrogen for divers at depth:

❏ A   it diffuses more rapidly into the body tissues
❏ B   it is denser
❏ C   it has a lower viscosity
❏ D   it has less narcotic effect
❏ E   it is a good insulator

1.69   In a recording of central venous pressure (CVP)

❏ A   the a wave is caused by atrial systole
❏ B   the c wave is caused by bulging of the tricuspid valve during isometric ventricular contraction
❏ C   the v wave is due to atrial filling when the tricuspid valve is closed
❏ D   the pressure wave is increased during inspiration
❏ E   the pressure wave is always raised if left atrial pressure is increased

1.70   Soda lime

- ❏   A   is mainly calcium carbonate
- ❏   B   can be used to scavenge nitrous oxide
- ❏   C   needs water to absorb carbon dioxide
- ❏   D   in a properly packed canister, half the volume should be space between granules
- ❏   E   gets hot in use

1.71   Warming blood to 37°C for massive blood transfusion

- ❏   A   reduces the incidence of infection
- ❏   B   increases the CO_2 tension
- ❏   C   reduces the O_2 tension
- ❏   D   shifts the O_2 dissociation curve to the right
- ❏   E   reduces the incidence of arrhythmias

1.72   Concerning fires and explosions in theatre

- ❏   A   the relative humidity in theatre should be about 66%
- ❏   B   air is safer than oxygen
- ❏   C   switches in the zone of risk should be spark proof
- ❏   D   the floor should be terrazzo on a well-conducting screed
- ❏   E   cotton fabrics are better than wool

1.73   Critical temperature

- ❏   A   of nitrous oxide is 36.5°C
- ❏   B   is the temperature below which a gas cannot be liquefied by pressure
- ❏   C   separates gases from vapours
- ❏   D   of O_2 is –182.5°C
- ❏   E   is always lower than the boiling point of the same gas

1.74   The following are true for gases in cylinders:

❏ A   nitrous oxide and entonox are filled to the same pressure
❏ B   a full oxygen cylinder is at a pressure of 1950 kPa
❏ C   nitrous oxide should contain 1% water vapour.
❏ D   nitrous oxide should not be stored below –8°C
❏ E   size E cylinders of oxygen and nitrous oxide are generally used on a Boyle's machine

1.75   With regard to pressure

❏ A   it is measured in Newtons
❏ B   it is defined as the force applied over a surface
❏ C   the absolute pressure of a cylinder of O_2 is 138 bar
❏ D   arterial blood pressure readings are gauge pressures
❏ E   when using a narrow capillary tube filled with water to measure pressure, the reading will be decreased due to the effect of surface tension

1.76   Regarding turbulent flow

❏ A   the flow is directly proportional to pressure
❏ B   the flow is directly proportional to the density of the fluid
❏ C   its onset can be predicted by a Reynolds' number greater than 1000
❏ D   warming anaesthetic gases increases the likelihood of turbulent flow
❏ E   this is more likely in the lower respiratory tract

1.77   Regarding the gas laws

❏   A   at constant temperature, the volume of a given mass of gas varies directly with the absolute pressure

❏   B   at constant pressure, the volume of a given mass of gas varies directly with the temperature

❏   C   at a constant volume, the temperature of a given mass of gas varies directly with the absolute pressure

❏   D   in a mixture of gases, the partial pressure that each gas exerts is dependent on the constituent mixture

❏   E   alteration of the state of a gas without allowing the temperature to alter, is known as an antidiabetic change

1.78   The critical temperature

❏   A   is the temperature below which a substance cannot be liquefied by pressure alone

❏   B   of oxygen is −119°C

❏   C   of nitrous oxide is 36.5°C

❏   D   applies only to a single gas; not a mixture

❏   E   of CO_2 is 31°C

1.79   Concerning humidification

❏   A   inspired gases in the trachea contain approximately 3 mg of water vapour per litre of dry gas, if dry gas has been inhaled

❏   B   of inspired gases results in less heat loss than warming inspired gases

❏   C   the heat moisture exchanger (HME) can give a humidity of the inspired gases of about 20 g/m^3

❏   D   the HME is more efficient and more effective as the ambient temperature increases

❏   E   using the HME can increase the work of breathing

1.80 **The following can be used for the measurement of temperature:**

❑ A the Seebeck effect
❑ B alcohol thermometers
❑ C mercury thermometers
❑ D resistance
❑ E interferometer

1.81 **A Wright's respirometer will give a reading which is lower than the actual value when there is**

❑ A low flow of gas
❑ B 30% oxygen in the gas
❑ C nitrous oxide present
❑ D humidity in the respirometer
❑ E an intermittent flow of gas

1.82 **Evoked potential techniques for measuring depth of anaesthesia utilise the following stimuli:**

❑ A auditory
❑ B oesophageal contractions
❑ C somatosensory
❑ D visual
❑ E magnetic resonance

1.83 **In exponential change**

❑ A the time constant is the time taken for the initial response to fall to half its value
❑ B in one time constant, 37% change is complete
❑ C in three time constants, 95% change is complete
❑ D the rate of change of a variable is proportional to the magnitude of the variable
❑ E the half-life is the time constant

1.84   Airway resistance

❑   A   can be measured by plethysmography
❑   B   is measured in kPa per litre
❑   C   increases during inhalation anaesthesia
❑   D   increases at high inspiratory flow rates
❑   E   decreases with the application of positive end expiratory
          pressure

1.85   The chances of microshock occurring increases due to

❑   A   saline filled catheters
❑   B   earth loop
❑   C   multiple earth connections
❑   D   isolated circuit
❑   E   oesophageal electrocardiogram

**1.86   The following are required to measure the cardiac output by
         the Fick principle:**

❑   A   arterial oxygen content
❑   B   venous oxygen content
❑   C   oxygen uptake
❑   D   respiratory quotient
❑   E   arterial carbon monoxide content

1.87   The Magill circuit

❑   A   is an example of a Mapleson A circuit
❑   B   is functionally similar to the Lack circuit
❑   C   is suitable for children over 25 kg
❑   D   is suitable for IPPV
❑   E   rebreathing and hypercarbia will occur if the fresh gas flow is
          less than the minute volume

1.88   Inaccuracies in the measurement of central venous pressure may arise from

❏   A   a change in the position of the patient
❏   B   misplacement of the catheter
❏   C   wetting of the cotton wool plug in the top of the manometer tube
❏   D   straining during respiration
❏   E   arterial hypotension

1.89   The accuracy of a rotameter may be affected by

❏   A   dirt on the bobbin
❏   B   static electricity
❏   C   passing the wrong gas through it
❏   D   back pressure from the Manley ventilator
❏   E   using it at high altitude

1.90   Capnography

❏   A   works on the absorption of carbon dioxide in the ultra violet region of the spectrum
❏   B   can be helpful in detecting air embolism before cardiovascular compromise occurs.
❏   C   the $PaCO_2/PeCO_2$ gradient in a patient with V/Q mismatch is 0.7 kPa
❏   D   collision broadening may occur in the presence of oxygen
❏   E   the two sampling methods are side and main stream

16 Stations: time allowed approximately 2 hours.

STATION 1.1

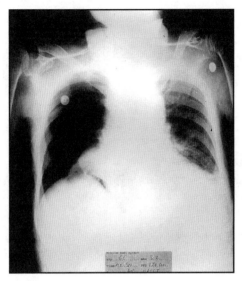

Fig. 1.1

(a) What is your diagnosis?

(b) Is this an AP or PA film? How do you know?

(c) What are the advantages of a PA film?

(d) Is there any rotation? How can you tell?

(e) Name 3 clinical signs one might expect to find in this patient.

(f) How would you manage this?

STATION 1.2

Please state whether the following statements regarding the electro-cardiograph shown below are **True** or **False**.

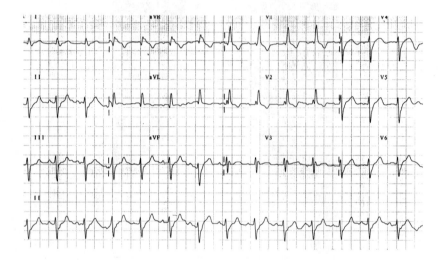

Fig. 1.2

	True	False
(a) The rate is normal	❑	❑
(b) The axis is normal	❑	❑
(c) The calibration is 1 mV/cm	❑	❑
(d) There is a right bundle branch block	❑	❑
(e) The patient has not had an acute myocardial infarction	❑	❑
(f) There is a bifascicular block pattern	❑	❑
(g) The patient needs a pacing wire	❑	❑
(h) There is a strong possibility of the patient developing complete heart block	❑	❑
(i) Anaesthesia is safe in this individual	❑	❑

STATION 1.3

You have a ventilated patient on the ITU with the following blood results:

Hb 8.7	INR 2.4	pH 7.15	HCO_3 15.3
WCC 2.7	APTT 2.1	pCO_2 6.1	BE -8.2
Plt 43	Fibrinogen 0.4	pO_2 9.6	FiO_2 0.7

He is in septic shock due to faecal peritonitis.

(a) What is the likely haematological problem visible on his results? Why?

(b) How would you manage this?

(c) What is abnormal about his arterial blood gases?

(d) Does he have any respiratory problems?

(e) How do you know?

(f) If the patient has not yet been operated on, is it safe to operate on him if he has been stabilised?

(g) What problems would be associated with anaesthesia?

STATION 1.4

There is a 54-year-old male alcoholic on the general medical ward with the following blood results:

Na	132	Protein	32
K	6.1	Alb	13
Urea	27.4		
Creat	533	Bili	447
HCO_3	17		

(a) What other tests would you consider as essential now?

(b) What would you expect the results to show?

(c) What is the probable cause of his raised urea and creatinine?

(d) Would you anaesthetise him for an acute abdomen? Why/why not?

(e) Is this likely to improve spontaneously without specialist intervention?

STATION 1.5

You have a 72-year-old gentleman on your list for an inguinal hernia repair. He is known to have ischaemic heart disease. Please obtain a relevant history from him.

STATION 1.6

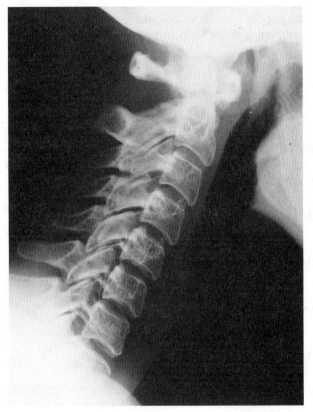

Fig. 1.6

(a) What does this X-ray show?

(b) What is its relevance to anaesthesia?

STATION 1.7

A 60-year-old lady with severe symptomatic oesophageal reflux needs surgery for varicose veins.

(a) What premedication will you prescribe and why?

(b) What sort of induction will you perform?

31

STATION 1.8

A 26-year-old woman is brought to the Accident and Emergency Department with the following blood gases:

pH	7.25
$PaCO_2$	3.6kPa
PaO_2	12.5 kPa
BE	-6.5

She complains of tinnitus and epigastric discomfort, but is reluctant to give much history. Her boyfriend suggests that she may have taken an overdose of some tablets.

(a) What is the diagnosis?

(b) How do you explain the arterial blood gases?

(c) How would you manage her?

STATION 1.9

You have a very anxious mother, who is a solicitor, in front of you. Her fit 5-year-old son is scheduled for a circumcision. She is very confrontational. Explain your choice of anaesthesia and analgesia to her, as well as possible alternatives. She does not like the idea of a caudal epidural injection or rectal medication. Reason with her why these are good options.

STATION 1.10

An adult male collapses behind you in the queue at a DIY store.

(a) Describe your actions, considering he remains unresponsive.

An ambulance eventually arrives. An ECG is attached, and you see the following rhythm:

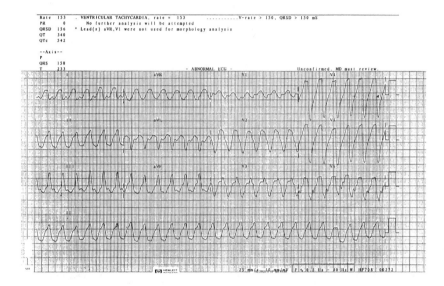

Fig. 1.10

(b) What would you do now?

STATION 1.11

(a) Is it true that central venous catheters are excellent for the rapid administration of intravenous fluids?

(b) What properties does the ideal cannula need for rapid fluid administration?

STATION 1.12

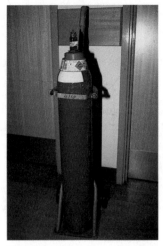

Fig.1.12

(a) What gas is contained in this cylinder?

(b) It is a mixture of what?

(c) What are the critical temperatures of the separate gases?

(d) What is the critical temperatures of the mixture?

(e) What happens if a full cylinder is allowed to cool below this temperature, and what clinical relevance does it have?

STATION 1.13

Decribe how you would insert a central venous catheter via the internal jugular route.

(a) What are the advantages of this route over the subclavian route?

(b) What are the potential complications of CVP line insertion and what steps would you take to minimise these?

STATION 1.14

You have been called to the labour ward, where a lady is having a convulsion post partum.

(a) What is the differential diagnosis?

(b) How would you manage her?

STATION 1.15

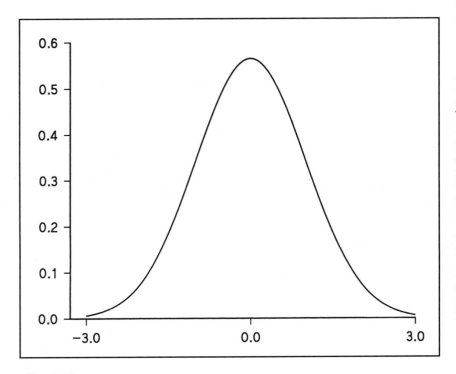

Fig. 1.15

(a) What is the above statistical curve called?

(b) What type of data does it represent?

(c) Are the mean, median and mode represented by the same point?

(d) If we are measuring pain scores in a different study, would Student's t-test be a good statistical test? Why/why not?

STATION 1.16

Explain cricoid pressure to a trainee ODP, who has never heard of it before.

Viva 1a

PHARMACOLOGY
Muscle relaxants

What types of muscle relaxants do you know?

What are the differences between the two groups?

How does a depolarising muscle relaxant work? Name two.

What is the principle behind the speed of onset of non-depolarising muscle relaxants?

What can you tell me about rocuronium?

PHYSIOLOGY
Inotropes

What is an inotrope?

Classify inotropes.

Discuss dopexamine.

Viva 1b

CLINICAL

This is an elderly lady who needs an urgent operation but has major intercurrent medical problems. She has a history of cardiac and cerebrovascular disease and on examination is confused, in atrial fibrillation and has signs of mitral regurgitation. Blood results show she is anti-coagulated (though not in fact adequately for a prosthetic heart valve) and also has a degree of renal impairment.

How would you anaesthetise her?

What are the options for post-operative analgesia?

PHYSICS
Laminar vs turbulent flow

Compare laminar and turbulent flow.

Do you have any equations explaining these? What is the Reynolds' number?

Are there any pieces of equipment based on the principle of laminar flow?

Explain how a pneumotachograph works.

MCQ PAPER 1 – ANSWERS

1.1   **Answers: C E**

Dopamine is both a catecholamine and a neurotransmitter. It is positively inotropic and chronotropic and may cause tachyarrhythmias. It causes renal artery dilatation. Dopamine is also an important neurotransmitter in the central nervous system, particularly in the basal ganglia. A deficiency of dopaminergic neurones in the basal ganglia causes Parkinsonism. Dopamine acts to inhibit prolactin secretion by the posterior pituitary gland. Finally, dopamine is the neurotransmitter at the chemoreceptor trigger zone. From the above information, it can be deduced that dopamine antagonists might cause extrapyramidal effects such as Parkinsonism and oculogyric crises. They may cause hyperprolactinaemia. Their principal use is as anti-emetics. The commonly encountered dopamine antagonists include the phenothiazines such as prochlorperazine and chlorpromazine, the butyrophenones such as haloperidol, droperidol and others such as metaclopramide.

As well as its anti-emetic effects, metoclopramide usefully raises lower oesophageal sphincter tone and promotes gastric emptying. These effects are due to cholinergic (not anti-dopaminergic) effects, however. Metoclopramide also has anti-serotoninergic effects.

1.2   **Answers: C D E**

Diamorphine is diacetyl morphine, it is rapidly metabolised in the liver to the active metabolites monoacetylmorphine and, ultimately, morphine. It is therefore a pro-drug with a high first pass metabolism. It is about twice as potent as morphine and is more rapid in action because of greater lipid solubility. Diamorphine is more euphoric and a better antitussive than morphine.

1.3   **Answers: D E**

Alfentanil is about one tenth as potent as fentanyl. The pKa of alfentanil is 6.5, whereas that of fentanyl is 8.4. Thus, at physiological pH, 89% of alfentanil is in the unionised form, whilst only 9% of fentanyl is unionised. Since it is the unionised form that crosses cell membranes, alfentanil acts much faster than fentanyl, despite being less lipid soluble. Alfentanil has a smaller volume of distribution and a shorter elimination half-life, and its duration of action is thus shorter than fentanyl. Alfentanil has minimal cardiovascular effects, although it may cause bradycardia and hypotension. Both drugs may cause muscle chest wall rigidity which may be so severe as to make artificial ventilation very difficult.

1.4   **Answers: B D**

Methohexitone is a methylated oxybarbiturate; the drug is reconstituted to make a 1% solution (10 mg/ml) which has a pH of 11. It is used mainly in electroconvulsive therapy and dental anaesthesia. Although it is a barbiturate, it may cause convulsions in epileptics and may precipitate porphyria. The usual dose in an adult is 1–2 mg/kg compared with 3–6 mg/kg for thiopentone. Both methohexitone and thiopentone are 80% bound to plasma proteins.

1.5   **Answers: A B E**

Propofol is 2,6,disopropylphenol. It is presented as a 1% white emulsion (10 mg/ml). The emulsion consists of 10% soya bean oil, 1.2% purified egg phosphatide and 2.25% glycerol. Propofol causes greater hypotension than thiopentone, mainly by vasodilatation, it also causes greater respiratory depression than thiopentone. The induction dose in an adult is 1.5–2.5 mg/kg. It is metabolised in the liver and other extra-hepatic sites such as the lungs.

1.6   **Answers: B C E**

Non-depolarising neuromuscular block is characterised by fade and post-tetanic facilitation, whilst fasciculations occur with the depolarising drugs such as suxamethonium. Non-depolarising muscle relaxant drugs are reversed by acetylcholinesterase inhibitors such as neostigmine. Neostigmine exacerbates block by a depolarising agent. The effects of non-depolarising agents are prolonged by hypothermia, hypokalaemia, hypocalcaemia and hypermagnesaemia, aminoglycosides and myasthenia gravis. Metabolic acidosis prolongs the effect of some, but not all, non-depolarising muscle relaxants.

1.7   **Answers: A B C E**

Atracurium is a non-depolarising muscle relaxant of the benzyl-isoquinolinium group. The other main group of relaxant drugs is the aminosteroids which include vecuronium. Atracurium is a mixture of ten isomers. Cis-atracurium is the R-cis R^{1}cis isomer of atracurium. Atracurium comes as a 1% solution (10 mg/ml), the adult dose is about 0.5 mg/kg. Atracurium is broken down by Hoffman degradation (which is temperature dependent) and alkaline ester hydrolysis. The former reaction produces laudanosine which causes seizures in dogs but seems harmless to humans. Hypothermia and acidosis prolong the action of atracurium. Atracurium can cause histamine release.

1.8   **Answers: A E**

Inotropic agents increase the force of contraction of the myocardium. Such agents include the catecholamines (such as dopamine, adrenaline and noradrenaline) which act by stimulating β-adrenergic receptors in the myocardium. Phosphodiesterase inhibitors (such as the theophyllines) act by blocking the breakdown of cAMP. cAMP is the second messenger which is produced by β-adrenergic receptor stimulation.

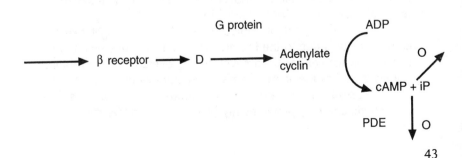

Glucagon is a positive inotrope which acts by stimulating the activity of adenylate cyclase, leading to an increase in intracellular concentrations of cAMP. Verapamil, propanolol and potassium all have negative inotropic effects.

1.9   **Answers: A D E**

Many drugs are metabolised in the liver. The cytochrome P450 enzyme system is the major metabolic route. Most drugs are metabolised to more water-soluble compounds which can then be renally excreted.

Hepatic metabolism usually involves two steps:

phase 1– oxidation, reduction, hydrolysis (cytochrome P450)

phase 2– conjugation with either glucuronide or by glycine, glutathione, sulphate, acetyl or methyl groups

1.10   **Answers: A B C D E**

Bupivacaine is an amide local anaesthetic agent. All amides have the same basic structure:

Bupivacaine has a longer duration of action than lignocaine and is more potent (0.25% bupivacaine is equipotent with 1% lignocaine). Bupivacaine is cardiotoxic and is contraindicated in intravenous regional anaesthesia (IVRA; Bier's block).

Prilocaine is the agent of choice for IVRA. It is thought that the cardiotoxicity is due to the D stereoisomer. The pure L enantiomer (laevobupivacaine) has been developed to overcome this problem. Ropivacaine has the same chemical structure as bupivacaine, but has one extra carbon atom in the amine R^1 group. It is less cardiotoxic and may preferentially block sensory rather than motor fibres.

1.11   **Answers: A B D**

1.12   **Answers: B C E**
The cytochrome P450 enzyme system is found in the endoplasmic recticulum of hepatocytes and is responsible for phase 1 metabolic reactions such as oxidation and reduction. The enzyme system can be induced or inhibited by drugs. Enzyme induction can lead to reduced plasma levels of drugs which undergo hepatic cytochrome P450 metabolism leading to a reduced pharmacological effect. Rifampicin is an enzyme inducing agent which may reduce the efficacy of drugs e.g. warfarin or the oral contraceptive pill which undergo hepatic cytochrome P450 metabolism. Conversely, inhibition of cytochrome P450 (by cimetidine for example) can lead to toxic levels of drugs such as phenytoin or warfarin.

P450	<u>induction</u>	<u>inhibition</u>
	barbiturates	cimetidine
	rifampicin	
	phenytoin &	
	other anticonvulsants	

1.13   **Answers: A B**
Midazolam is presented as a solution with a pH < 4. On entering venous blood, the pH increases and the structure of the molecule changes in such a way as to render it active. Atracurium undergoes spontaneous Hoffman degradation (which is both temperature and pH dependent). Its structure changes with pH.

1.14   **Answers: A C D**
Metoclopramide is a dopamine antagonist which is used as an anti-emetic.
It also raises lower oesophageal sphincter tone. Like other anti-dopaminergic drugs, it may cause extrapyramidal effects such as oculogyric crises, especially in the young.
Since dopamine is a prolactin inhibiting factor, drugs which are anti-dopaminergic can cause hyperprolactinaemia.

1.15   **Answers: A B C**

Uterine smooth muscle has sympathetic and parasympathetic innervation. Sympathetic stimulation by β_2-adrenoreceptor agonists such as salbutamol or ritodrine relaxes the uterus; whilst parasympathetic stimulation causes contraction. Neostigmine, by inhibiting acetylcholinesterase, has parasympathomimetic effects. Amyl nitrate and halothane directly relax smooth muscle. Oxytocin and its analogue are potent uterine contractors.

1.16   **Answers: A B C**

The rate of transfer of a molecule across the placenta is indirectly proportional to its size and directly related to its lipid solubility. Clearly, the blood flow to the placenta is important too.

1.17   **Answers: A C D**

All the volatile agents cause a reduction in cerebrovascular resistance. Thiopentone and fentanyl cause little change.

1.18   **Answers: A B C**

Nitrous oxide (N_2O) may be contaminated by nitric oxide (NO) and nitrogen dioxide (NO_2) produced during the manufacture of nitrous oxide. The higher oxides of nitrogen can produce pulmonary oedema several hours after inhalation, and pulmonary fibrosis 2–3 weeks later. They may also cause methaemoglobinaemia. N_2O is manufactured by heating ammonium nitrate to 240°C. Ammonia is produced in this reaction and may contaminate nitrous oxide. It too can cause pulmonary oedema.

1.19   **Answer: C**

Nifedipine is a calcium channel blocking drug used to treat hypertension. It is a vasodilator, causing a drop in cardiac output, hypotension and reflex tachycardia. It may be taken orally or sublingually and may cause headache, flushing, dizziness and peripheral oedema.

1.20   Answers: **B D**

Ropivacaine is a new amide local anaesthetic agent. It is less potent than bupivacaine, but has a similar duration of action. It causes less central nervous system and cardiovascular toxicity than bupivacaine, and, in addition, less motor block. It is presented as the pure S enantiomer, not a racemic mixture. Bupivacaine is a racemic mixture, but should also soon be available commercially as the pure enantiomer. The pKa of ropivacaine and bupivacaine are identical.

1.21   Answers: **A B D**

Magnesium is the second most plentiful intracellular cation after potassium, and is one of the most important regulators of intracellular biochemistry. The normal plasma level is 0.75–1.0 mmol/l. Magnesium is used therapeutically to control cardiac arrhythmias and as an anticonvulsant in eclampsia. Magnesium toxicity causes neuromuscular blockade by inhibiting acetylcholine release at the neuromuscular junction. The primary clinical manifestation of this is respiratory depression and loss of tendon reflexes. Treatment is intravenous calcium gluconate. Magnesium is controlled by parathormone, but not by calcitonin.

1.22   Answers: **A B C D E**

Isoflurane causes a small (10%) drop in cardiac output in healthy volunteers, mainly by a decrease in stroke volume. Isoflurane causes significant peripheral vasodilatation and hypotension with a reflex compensatory tachycardia.

1.23   Answers: **B D E**

Propofol is presented as a white aqueous emulsion containing 10% soya bean oil, 2.25% glycerol and 1.2% purified egg phosphatide. It has a pH of 7 and a pKa of 11. It causes more respiratory depression and greater hypotension than thiopentone. It is metabolised in the liver as well as at other extra-hepatic sites.

1.24   Answers: **A B C E**

Benzodiazepines and barbiturates are anticonvulsants. Chlormethiazole and ethosuximide are also anticonvulsants.

1.25   **Answer: A**

Suxamethonium is a depolarising neuromuscular blocking agent. It
is stored at 4°C in the fridge; although its potency in fact decreases
very slowly if left at room temperature. Chemically, suxamethonium
is 2 molecules of acetylcholine linked by ester bonds. The ester
bonds are broken down by plasma cholinesterase. The productivity
of this enzyme is controlled genetically by at least five alleles. A
proportion of the population have atypical plasma cholinesterase
and metabolise the drug more slowly than normal. Low levels of
plasma cholinesterase are found in patients undergoing plasmapheresis, in liver failure, in malnutrition, during pregnancy, and in
patients taking the oral contraceptive pill, lithium or
cyclophosphamide. The side-effects of suxamethonium include:
hyperkalaemia, muscle pains and bradycardia; especially with
repeat doses. Suxamethonium may be given i.m. (intramuscularly)
but it is painful.

1.26   **Answers: A D**

Vecuronium is a non-depolarising muscle relaxant. It is a
monoquaternary aminosteroid. It acts in about 2 minutes and has a
duration of action of about 20–30 minutes. It is devoid of
cardiovascular actions and is metabolised in the liver to inactive
products.

1.27   **Answers: B D**

Ketamine is a phencyclidine derivative. It produces a state known
as dissociative anaesthesia. Its mode of action includes antagonism
at the N-methyl-D-aspartate (NMDA) receptor as well as actions at
the adrenergic, cholinergic, serotoninergic and opioid receptors. It
is a potent analgesic as well as being a bronchodilator and
sympathomimetic agent. It is thus useful in asthmatic and shocked
patients, but contraindicated in angina and hypertension. It causes
hypersalivation and increased bronchial secretions. An anti-
sialogogue pre-medication is often therefore used with ketamine. It
raises intraocular and intracranial pressure and may produce
disturbing emergence reactions. It undergoes hepatic metabolism
and renal excretion; only 2.5% is excreted unchanged in the urine.

1.28   **Answer: E**

Atenolol is a relatively selective antagonist at the β_1-receptors. Despite this, it is not entirely safe in asthmatics as blockade of β_2-receptors may precipitate bronchospasm. Like all beta blockers, atenolol is a negative inotrope and may be unsafe in diabetics as it may mask the sympathetic symptoms of hypoglycaemia, such as sweating and tachycardia. Atenolol is renally excreted and should not be used in patients with renal failure as it will accumulate.

1.29   **Answers: C E**

Lignocaine is an amide local anaesthetic which is highly protein bound (65%). It undergoes hepatic metabolism by amidases; unlike the ester local anaesthetics, such as cocaine, which are degraded by plasma cholinesterase. It undergoes extensive first pass metabolism (70%). The half-life of lignocaine is increased in haemorrhagic shock because of reduced hepatic blood flow, and therefore a reduced rate of metabolism.

1.30   **Answers: C D**

Amiodarone is in class III of the Vaughan-Williams' classification of anti-arrhythmics. It is used to treat both ventricular and supraventricular arrhythmias. It has a number of side-effects, including a photosensitive slate-grey skin discoloration and reversible corneal microdeposits. It is an iodine containing compound, and can therefore interfere with thyroid function. It can cause hypo- or hyperthyroidism. It can cause pulmonary fibrosis, hepatic dysfunction and peripheral neuropathy. It has a very long half-life.

1.31   **Answers: D E**

Hypercalcaemia occurs in hyperparathyroidism. Hypocalcaemia occurs in hypoparathyroidism and also in acute pancreatitis. Hyperglycaemia is seen in phaeochromocytoma due to high levels of catecholamines. Malignant hyperpyrexia leads to muscle breakdown, release of intracellular potassium and hyperkalaemia. The TURP syndrome is caused by excessive absorption of irrigation fluid into the vascular space and leads to hyponatraemia.

1.32   **Answer: All false**

In pregnancy, there are great physiological changes.

- The circulation is hyperdynamic with a reduced systemic vascular resistance and an increase in heart rate, stroke volume and cardiac output.
- Although there is an increase in red cell mass, there is an even greater increase in plasma volume leading to the physiological anaemia of pregnancy.
- The oxygen dissociation curve shifts to the right, thus facilitating oxygen uptake by the fetal red cells.
- In the respiratory system, there is a reduction in functional residual capacity, but an increased tidal volume and respiratory rate.
- There is an increase in fibrinogen and reduced fibrinolysis leading to a hypercoagulable state.
- The lower oesophageal sphincter tone is reduced in pregnancy leading to an increased likelihood of gastric reflux. It is because of this that pregnant women having a general anaesthetic are given sodium citrate and ranitidine and have a rapid sequence induction with cricoid pressure to reduce the chance of regurgitation and aspiration of acidic stomach contents.

1.33   **Answer: C**

Bleeding is unlikely until the platelet count falls to 50 x 10^9/l and may not occur until an even lower level. Haemophilia is an X-linked disorder in which there is a deficiency of factor VIII. It results in a prolongation of the APTT. The PT, platelet count and bleeding time are all normal. Stored blood contains no functional platelets and is deficient in the labile clotting factors (factors V and VIII). Multiple transfusions therefore lead to a coagulopathy. Most of the clotting factors are synthesised in the liver, although only factors 2, 7, 9 and 10 are dependent on vitamin K for their synthesis. In someone who is bleeding because of excessive warfarin administration, only fresh frozen plasma (FFP) will rapidly reverse the effect of warfarin. Vitamin K will act more slowly and, in addition, prevents re-anticoagulation with warfarin for up to a week.

1.34   **Answers: B C**

The treatment of pulmonary embolism is i.v. heparin and warfarin in the longer term. Thrombolytic therapy (e.g. streptokinase) is generally reserved for large pulmonary emboli in which there is evidence of right ventricular compromise. Operations involving the knee, hip and pelvis are most commonly associated with DVT. Regional anaesthesia on patients receiving prophylactic subcutaneous heparin is controversial. However, several large surveys have shown no increase in incidence of haematoma formation. HRT and low oestrogen/progesterone oral contraceptives are not associated with an increased incidence of deep venous thrombosis.

1.35   **Answers: A B C**

The blood gases reveal hypoxia and respiratory alkalosis from hyperventilation; type 1 respiratory failure. This could be due to altitude. At sea level, barometric pressure is 100 kPa and air contains 21% oxygen. The partial pressure of oxygen being inspired is therefore 21 kPa. At 5,500 metres, for example, the barometric pressure is about 50 kPa, so the partial pressure of oxygen being inspired is only about 10 kPa The arterial oxygen tension might be expected, therefore, to be about 8 kPa. Hypoxic stimulation of the peripheral chemoreceptors causes hyperventilation and a respiratory alkalosis. A pneumothorax, if large enough, can cause hypoxia as blood passes through the non-ventilated lung causing a shunt. The hypoxia stimulates ventilation and the $PaCO_2$ is lowered. However, in most small spontaneous pneumothoraces, the blood gases are normal. In hysteria, there is hyperventilation and a resultant respiratory alkalosis, but the $PaCO_2$ will be normal. Salicylate poisoning initially causes hyperventilation and a respiratory alkalosis due to direct stimulation of the respiratory centre. In severe overdose, there is uncoupling of oxidative phosphorylation and a metabolic acidosis. Carbon monoxide (CO) has an affinity for oxygen 240 times that of haemoglobin. Thus, in CO poisoning, there is usually a reduced PaO_2 and compensatory hyperventilation.

1.36

Answers: A E

Acute hypovolaemia causes a release of catecholamines leading to tachycardia and vasoconstriction. The blood flow to essential organs such as kidneys and brain is preserved unless the hypovolaemia is severe. There is activation of the compensatory ADH and renin-angiotensin-aldosterone systems leading to salt and water retention. The PaO_2 and $PaCO_2$ are generally unchanged. There may be an increase in physiological dead space as areas of lung may be underperfused, and as a result, an increased alveolar to arterial oxygen gradient.

1.37

Answers: A B C D

Platelets are necessary for clot retraction to occur; clot retraction is caused by platelet contractile microfilaments. Contraction of the microfilaments is activated by calcium ions (released from stores in the mitochondria and endoplasmic reticulum) and thrombin (precursor prothrombin). In order to form a clot a platelet plug must be bound by fibrin which is formed by the action of thrombin on fibrinogen.

1.38

Answers: A B C D E

An increase in $PaCO_2$ leads to release of catecholamines from the adrenal medulla and the resulting sympathetic overactivity is manifested as tachycardia, hypertension, sweating and mydriasis. Hypercarbia also causes narcosis and unconsciousness.

1.39

Answers: A B D E

A Valsalva manoeuvre is a forced expiration against a closed glottis. This leads to a raised intrathoracic pressure The initial effect is a transient increase in blood pressure as blood is squeezed out of the thorax and into the systemic circulation. There is then, however, a reduction in venous return to the right side of the heart, leading to a reduction in stroke volume, cardiac output and blood pressure. The baroreceptor mediated compensation causes a tachycardia and increased peripheral vascular resistance. Once the manoeuvre is terminated, the venous return is restored and the blood pressure rises transiently to a level greater than normal. A baroreceptor mediated bradycardia occurs at this stage.

1.40   **Answers: A D E**

Albumin has a molecular weight of about 65,000 Daltons. It is synthesised in the liver, and is therefore reduced in liver disease. Malabsorption leads to reduced absorption of the amino acids necessary for albumin synthesis. The normal serum albumin concentration is 35–50 g/l. Albumin exerts several effects including: maintenance of colloid osmotic pressure, free radical scavenging and binding and transport of drugs.

1.41   **Answers: A E**

The metabolic rate decreases during sleep and hypothermia. Tidal volume decreases with deepening levels of sleep. Respiratory rate increases slightly in all stages of sleep but the minute volume is progressively reduced in parallel with the tidal volume. The minute volume is increased by an increase in body acidity to create a compensatory respiratory alkalosis by removing carbon dioxide from the body.

At high altitude the decrease in inspired gas pO_2 reduces alveolar and therefore arterial pO_2. The actual decrease in alveolar pO_2 is tempered by hyperventilation caused by the hypoxic drive to ventilation.

1.42   **Answers: A B C E**

The oxyhaemoglobin dissociation curve is moved to the right (the Bohr effect) by an increase in temperature, hydrogen ion concentration (lowered pH, acidosis) and 2,3-diphosphoglycerate (2,3-DPG). Anaemia is associated with an increase in 2,3-DPG, and therefore a right shift of the curve. A shift of the curve to the right facilitates oxygen delivery to the tissues.

1.43   **Answers: D E**

Blood returning to the right side of the heart has an oxygen saturation of about 75%; the tissues having extracted about 25% of the oxygen delivered to them. Blood is then pumped through the pulmonary artery and is oxygenated as it passes through the lungs before returning to the left atrium via the pulmonary veins. The pressures in the heart are :

right atrium	5 mmHg
right ventricle	25/5 mmHg
pulmonary artery	25/10 mmHg
left atrium	8 mmHg
left ventricle	125/8 mmHg

1.44   **Answer: C**

The autonomic nervous system consists of sympathetic and parasympathetic systems. The neurotransmitter at all autonomic ganglia is acetylcholine (ACH). All preganglionic fibres (sympathetic or parasympathetic) release ACH including fibres which supply the chromaffin cells of the adrenal medulla. The neurotransmitter at the post-ganglionic nerve endings is ACH for the parasympathetic system and noradrenaline for the sympathetic system; except sympathetic fibres to sweat glands which produce ACH.

1.45   **Answers: B D E**

Sodium reabsorption in the kidney is mainly under the influence of the renin–angiotensin–aldosterone system. Renin is produced by the juxtaglomerular apparatus of the kidney in response to reduced blood flow or hyponatraemia. Renin circulates in the blood and acts on angiotensinogen, produced by the lungs, converting it to angiotensin. Angiotensin acts as a vasoconstrictor and stimulates production of aldosterone by the adrenal cortex. Aldosterone acts on the proximal tubules of the kidney to promote sodium reabsorption. Antidiuretic hormone (ADH) is produced by the posterior pituitary and acts on the collecting ducts to promote water reabsorption. The loop of Henle acts to produce a hypertonic renal medulla. This involves active chloride, but passive sodium reabsorption.

1.46   **Answers: A B C D E**

Block of the cervical sympathetic ganglia leads to Horner's syndrome which is characterised by miosis, enophthalmos, anhidrosis, nasal congestion, ptosis and dilatation of conjunctival vessels.

1.47   **Answers: A C D E**

Metabolic acidosis is either caused by ingestion or production of excess acid (e.g. salicylate poisoning or diabetic ketoacidosis) or by either failure to excrete acid or excessive loss of bicarbonate (e.g. renal failure or diarrhoea). Transplantation of the ureters into the colon causes a hyperchloraemic acidosis.

1.48 Answers: B C D E

Pyloric stenosis causes vomiting of acidic stomach contents (hydrogen and chloride ions) without loss of the alkaline small bowel contents. Thus, a metabolic alkalosis with hypochloraemia ensues. The body attempts to compensate for metabolic alkalosis by hypoventilation and by renal retention of hydrogen ions. However vomiting also leads to hypovolaemia and dehydration and correction of this takes precedence over correction of acid base status. Thus the kidney paradoxically produces potassium and acid urine by excreting hydrogen ions in exchange for sodium and water. Thus the metabolic alkalosis is exacerbated and in addition hypokalemia produced.

1.49 Answers: A B C E

Red blood cells contains a number of surface antigens. The ABO and Rhesus are two separate systems which are used to type red cells and avoid haemolytic transfusion reactions.

The following table shows how the how the ABO system works.

Blood group	Red cell antigens	Antibodies
A	A	Anti-B
B	B	Anti-A
AB	A + B	None
O	None	Anti-A/Anti-B

With the Rhesus system, a person who is Rhesus positive expresses the Rhesus antigen on red cells; a Rhesus negative person has no Rhesus antigen on the red cells. A person who is blood group O Rhesus negative thus has neither ABO nor Rhesus antigens and is a universal donor. Other less antigenic red cell surface antigens include Kell, Kidd and Duffy.

1.50 Answer: D

Intubation of the right main bronchus leads initially to elevated inflation pressure and hypoxaemia. At a later stage it may lead to collapse of the right upper lobe. There is no effect in the blood pressure nor is there hypercapnia.

1.51   **Answers: All false**

The normal arterial pH range is 7.35–7.45. A pH of 7.4 is equivalent to a hydrogen ion concentration of 40 nmol/L. With blood gas the measured parameters are PO_2, pCO_2 and pH. From these measurements, other parameters can be derived e.g. bicarbonate, base excess, oxygen content and oxygen saturation.

The arterial pH is maintained within narrow limits mainly by excretion of CO_2 by the lungs and to a lesser extent by excretion of hydrogen ions by the kidney (the bicarbonate system). The neonatal pH range is lower than that of the adult.

1.52   **Answer: B**

The time taken for the depolarisation wave to pass from the sinoatrial node, across the atria and through the atrioventricular node into ventricular muscle is called the PR interval. The normal PR interval is 0.12–0.2 seconds. The QT interval represents the total time taken by ventricular depolarisation and repolarisation. It is normally < 0.44 seconds. The QRS complex represents ventricular depolarisation and conduction delay is present when its duration is > 0.12 seconds. The T wave represents ventricular repolarisation. The ST interval is the transient period when no further electrical current can be passed through the myocardium.

1.53   **Answers: B C D E**

Dead space is the volume of inspired air that takes no part in gas exchange. It is made up of the volume of the conducting airways (anatomical dead space) and that part of the alveolar volume occupying alveoli which are inadequately perfused with blood and therefore not taking part in gas exchange (alveolar dead space). Physiological dead space equals anatomical dead space plus alveolar dead space. The anatomical dead space may be measured using Fowler's method. It is the physiological dead space which is derived from the Bohr equation. The FRC is the amount of gas remaining in the lungs at the end of a normal expiration (about 2.5 litres in an adult). It cannot be measured directly. It can be measured using the helium dilution method, or by a nitrogen washout technique or with a body plethysmograph.

1.54   **Answers: B C E**

The GFR is the volume of plasma (ml) filtered by the kidneys per minute. It is normally about 125 ml/min. GFR can be measured using the relationship GFR = UV/P (where U = urine concentration of substance, V = volume of urine produced per minute and P = concentration of substance in plasma) for any substance that is freely filtered and not reabsorbed or secreted. Inulin, a fructose polysaccharide, fulfills these criteria. Sodium reabsorption in the renal tubules leads to a low excretion rate and low urinary concentration of sodium.

1.55   **Answers: A E**

The basal metabolic rate (BMR) is the energy output per unit of time of an individual, determined at rest in a room at a comfortable temperature in the thermoneutral zone, 12–14 hours after the last meal. The BMR increases by 14% for every degree centigrade rise in body temperature. BMR is higher in males and children and decreases with age. Foods, especially protein, increase heat production by their 'specific dynamic action'. Most of this specific dynamic action is due to oxidative deamination of amino acids in the liver.

1.56   **Answer: D**

The best source of non-protein energy in parenteral nutrition is a balanced combination of carbohydrate and fat (usually 2/3 carbohydrate and 1/3 lipid). Glucose is the preferred intravenous carbohydrate source. It has been used in the past as the sole energy source but this has disadvantages; hyperglycaemia, fatty infiltration of the liver, excessive carbon dioxide production (requiring extra respiratory effort) and essential fatty acid deficiency. Nitrogen requirements are decreased in elderly, female, frail and starved patients. Factors which increase the nitrogen requirements are youth, male sex, large body frame, trauma and sepsis. The preferred choice of nitrogen for parenteral nutrition is a solution of L-amino acids. Glutamine is thought to play an important role in the maintenance of gut mucosal integrity.

1.57   **Answers: A B E**

The specific heat of blood and injectate is used in the calculations. The Fick technique is used to measure cardiac output and blood flow to individual organs and is based on the Fick principle. This states that the amount of a substance taken up by an organ (or the body) per unit time is equal to the blood flow multiplied by the difference in concentration of that substance between arterial and mixed venous blood. In practice, the average steady-state oxygen consumption ($\dot{V}O_2$) of the whole body is measured for about 15 minutes, during which time blood samples are taken from a systemic artery and pulmonary artery (mixed venous blood). The samples are then analysed for the oxygen content of arterial (CaO_2) and mixed venous ($C\dot{v}O_2$) blood and cardiac output ($\dot{Q}$) is calculated from:

$$\dot{Q}\,(L\ min^{-1}) = \dot{V}O_2\ (L\ min^{-1})\ /\ CaO_2 - C\dot{v}O_2\ \text{(litre of } O_2 \text{ per litre of blood)}$$

The thermodilution technique involves injecting a solution that is colder than blood through the right atrial port of a pulmonary artery catheter and measuring the temperature change distally with a thermistor. Cardiac output is proportional to this temperature change divided by the area under the temperature change against time curve. Pulmonary artery temperature variation occurs from right ventricle surface cooling from the overlying lung during panting, deep spontaneous respirations and with Valsalva manoeuvres.

1.58   **Answers: A B D**

The Glasgow Coma Scale consists of 3 categories with a score for each, totalled to give an overall score from 3 to 15.

Best motor response	Best verbal response	Eye opening
6 to command	5 fully orientated	4 spontaneous
5 localizes to pain	4 confused	3 to command
4 withdrawal to pain	3 inappropriate words	2 to pain
3 flexes to pain	2 incomprehensible	1 none
2 extends to pain	sounds	
1 no response	1 no response	

As with CVP readings, changes in scores over time are often more useful than single values. There is a modified Glasgow Coma Scale for children which provides helpful information.

1.59   **Answer: A**

1 mmHg = 1.4 cmH$_2$O or 1 cmH$_2$O = 0.76 mmHg.

The CVP is a good indicator of right ventricular preload and right ventricular function. The CVP is a reasonable indicator of left atrial pressure in patients with normal myocardial and pulmonary function. The pulmonary artery catheter is a more reliable monitor for left-sided pressures and performance. Ideally the catheter tip should lie in the superior vena cava above the pericardial reflection to reduce the risk of thrombi, arrhythmias and cardiac tamponade if erosion and bleeding occur. The CVP primarily reflects right-sided function, therefore CVP can be normal in the presence of left ventricular failure and pulmonary oedema or raised in right-sided failure with normal left-sided function. Venoconstriction increases the CVP.

1.60   **Answers: A E**

Pulsatile veins may cause the pulse oximeters to under read as the technique cannot tell the difference between pulsating veins and arterioles e.g. in tricuspid incompetence. The amount of transmitted light is sensed several hundred times per second to allow for precise estimation of the peak and trough of each pulse waveform. Pulse oximeters average their readings every 10–20 seconds so they cannot detect acute desaturation. They therefore give a comparatively late warning of, for example, failure of oxygen supply or oxygen failure. The light for measurement comes from light emitting diodes of wavelengths 660 nm and 940 nm.

For every 1% carboxyhaemoglobin circulating, the pulse oximeter over reads by about 1%. 50% of cigarette smokers have carboxyhaemoglobin levels of > 6%. Methaemoglobinaemia leads to a falsely low saturation. Other factors affecting the accuracy of pulse oximetry are methylene blue, indocyanine green, opaque nail varnish, extraneous light sources, peripheral vasoconstriction, excessive movement and drugs responsible for the production of methaemoglobinaemia e.g. EDTA, local anaesthetic agents.

1.61 **Answers: A C D**

The stoichiometric concentration of a fuel and oxidising agent is the concentration at which all the combustible vapour and agent are completely used. Therefore the most violent and fastest reactions occur in stoichiometric mixtures. The risk of explosion is greater at stoichiometric concentrations. Nitrous oxide supports combustion more fiercely than oxygen. Nitrous oxide breaks down to oxygen and nitrogen with heat and produces further energy; thus reactions may be more vigorous with nitrous oxide than with oxygen alone. 1 microjoule of energy is sufficient for reactions in oxygen while 100 microjoules are required with air. The risk of sparking is greater in cold, dry environments.

1.62 **Answers: B C**

The post-tetanic count is useful during periods of intense neuro-muscular blockade (when there is no response to train of four stimulation). A 50 Hz tetanic stimulus is applied for 5 seconds followed by a pause of 3 seconds; then the number of twitches produced by single pulses at 1 Hz is counted. If the count is 6 then the first reaction to train of four will occur in less than 10 minutes, if the count is only 2, the response will require 15 minutes or longer. Train of four stimulation consists of 4 supramaximal stimuli at 2 Hz. If large amounts of suxamethonium are used, dual block, in which features of a non-depolarising neuromuscular block gradually replace those of depolarising blockade, may supervene.

Use of the orbicularis oculi (facial nerve) underestimates the degree of neuromuscular blockade because of direct muscle stimulation and relative insensitivity of the facial muscles to neuromuscular blockers. This is in contrast to using abductor pollicis (ulnar nerve) which is more sensitive than the diaphragm and vocal cords to neuromuscular blockers.

1.63   **Answers: A B C E**

A sine wave pattern is used for cutting and a damped or pulsed sine wave pattern for coagulation. In bipolar diathermy the current passes from one blade of a pair of forceps to the other i.e. passes across the tissue held between the tips of a pair of forceps. The circuit is earth-free – no plate electrode is required. The current does not pass through any part of the patient's body other than that between the forceps. The power required is small and it is electrically safer than unipolar diathermy. However it is only suitable for the coagulation of small pieces of tissues or blood vessels e.g. in ophthalmic surgery or neurosurgery.

1.64   **Answer: C**

Maintaining an ambient temperature of 22–24°C and a humidity of 50–70% minimises heat loss. Giving cold fluids into a central vein decreases core temperature more rapidly than giving them peripherally. Phenothiazines have an alpha-adrenoceptor antagonist effect and therefore cause vasodilatation. Space blankets are made of shiny, reflective, metallised plastic foil and should not be used in theatre because of the increased risks of burns and electrical shock.

1.65   **Answers: B E**

The width of the cuff should be 20% greater than the diameter of the arm. Too narrow a cuff leads to falsely high blood pressure readings whereas too loose a cuff produces falsely low pressures. For accurate measurement of blood pressure, there should be a fast cuff inflation to avoid venous congestion and a slow deflation to allow enough time to detect the arterial pulsation. If the cuff pressure is released too quickly the pressure recorded tends to be erroneously low because of the delay between passing the real pressure and seeing the reading. The resistance to occlusion of the blood vessel wall by the cuff is increased in atherosclerosis.

1.66   **Answer: D**

The saturated vapour pressure (SVP) is not linearly related to temperature; it increases with temperature according to a complex equation which approximates to an exponential relation. When SVP equals atmospheric pressure, the liquid boils. SVP depends on the temperature and the nature of the liquid only. The SVP for water at body temperature is 6.3 kPa.

1.67　　　　　　　　　　　　　　　　　　　　**Answers: B D**

Flowrate is described by the Hageni–Poiseuille equation;

$$V = \frac{\Delta P \pi r^4}{8 l \mu}$$

Where V = rate of flow, P = pressure gradient along tube, r = radius of tube, μ = viscosity of fluid and l = length of tube.

1.68　　　　　　　　　　　　　　　　　　　　**Answer: D**

The problem of nitrogen narcosis can be avoided by breathing a helium/oxygen mixture rather than a nitrogen/oxygen mixture because helium is only half as soluble as nitrogen so that less is dissolved in the tissues. Helium is less dense than nitrogen which decreases gas flow resistance and therefore the work of breathing. Helium/oxygen mixtures have a greater viscosity than nitrogen/oxygen mixtures. This is why helium is of no use in lower airway obstruction (e.g. asthma) where flow is laminar and therefore depends on viscosity rather than density.

1.69　　　　　　　　　　　　　　　　　　　　**Answers: A B C**

End-inspiratory and end-expiratory values for CVP in healthy individuals are normally −5 and −3 cmH_2O, respectively. Right atrial pressures do not always reflect left atrial pressures; e.g. left ventricular failure or infarction, valvular heart disease.

1.70　　　　　　　　　　　　　　　　　　　　**Answers: C D E**

Soda lime contains 80% calcium hydroxide, 4% sodium hydroxide, 14–20% added water content and a pH indicator. The sodium hydroxide improves the reactivity of the mixture and has hygroscopic properties (binding the necessary added water in the mixture). The addition of silica to help form the required granule size is no longer needed in modern manufacturing processes. Potassium hydroxide, which was thought to improve the activity of soda lime when cold, is no longer added. The reaction of carbon dioxide with soda lime is an exothermic reaction; the temperature within the canister can reach 60°C.

1.71　　　　　　　　　　　　　　　　　　　　**Answers: C D E**

At 4°C, bacterial replication in blood is inhibited. An increase in temperature, acidosis, raised carbon dioxide level and increased 2,3-diphosphoglycerate levels shift the O_2 dissociation curve to the right. Rapid transfusion of cold blood can cause cardiac arrest; cold blood is arrhythmogenic.

1.72   **Answers: A B C D E**

The relative humidity in theatre should be 50–70%. This is a compromise. Too high a humidity is uncomfortable and tiring for the staff but a low humidity increases the risk of explosion due to static electricity. Air contains approximately 79% nitrogen and nitrogen does not support combustion. An explosive mixture with air requires about 100 microjoules of energy to ignite it; this is 100 times the energy required to ignite an explosive mixture with oxygen.

An area extending for 25 cm around any part of the anaesthetic circuit or gas paths of an anaesthetic apparatus should be regarded as a zone of risk (AAGBI 1971). It is the area of theatre where mixtures of anaesthetic agents may be explosive. Within the zone of risk there should be no naked flames, all electrical switches should be spark proof and all parts should be made of conductive (antistatic) materials. Antistatic rubber containing carbon has enough conductivity to remove static electricity, but sufficient resistance to prevent a spark occurring from too rapid a discharge. The floor is constructed of terrazzo screed which acts as a large capacitor. The resistance of the floor over a distance of 60 cm should be 20,000–5,000,000 Ω. This allows the slow discharge of current to earth. Wool and nylon readily acquire static charge.

1.73   **Answers: A C**

The critical temperature is the temperature above which a substance cannot be liquefied no matter how much pressure is applied. A vapour is a substance in the gaseous phase below its critical temperature i.e. its constituent particles may enter the liquid form. Strictly speaking a substance is a gas when at a temperature above its critical temperature. The critical temperature of oxygen is –118 °C.

1.74   **Answer: E**

Nitrous oxide is stored at a pressure of 44 bar (4400 kPa) as a liquid in equilibrium with its vapour. Entonox is stored at a pressure of 137 bar (13,700 kPa) as a gas. A full cylinder of oxygen is stored at 137 bar (13,700 kPa). Medical gases are supplied as dry gases to prevent corrosion, condensation and frost in cylinders, pipes or valves. Entonox should not be stored below its pseudocritical temperature of –6°C, the temperature at which it may separate out into its constituent parts (lamination).

1.75   Answers: B C D

Force is measured in Newtons. Pressure is the force applied or distributed over a surface i.e. force per unit area. The SI unit of pressure is the Pascal and 1 Pascal is a pressure of 1 Newton active over an area of 1 square metre (1 Pa = 1 N/m^2). Cylinders are normally calibrated in gauge pressure i.e. the pressure above atmospheric pressure. Absolute pressure = gauge pressure + atmospheric pressure (= 137 bar + 1 bar = 138 bar in the case of oxygen cylinders). The reading will be increased in the case of a water manometer and decreased in the case of a mercury manometer due to the effect of surface tension.

1.76   Answers: All false

Turbulent flow is directly proportional to both the radius of the orifice squared and the square root of pressure and inversely proportional to the square root of the density of the fluid.

Reynolds' number = density x velocity x diameter of tube/ viscosity.

If Reynolds' number exceeds 2000, turbulent flow is more likely. Warming gases decreases their density and increases their viscosity, thereby decreasing Reynolds' number and making turbulent flow less likely. Turbulent flow is more likely in the trachea. In the bronchial tree, flow is mainly transitional and true laminar flow probably only occurs in the very small airways.

1.77   Answers: B C

Boyle's Law: At constant temperature, the volume of a given mass of gas varies inversely with the absolute pressure.
Charles' Law: At constant pressure, the volume of a given mass of gas varies directly with the absolute temperature.
Third Gas Law: At constant volume, the absolute pressure of a given mass of gas varies directly with temperature.
Dalton's Law of Partial Pressures: In a mixture of gases the pressure exerted by each gas is the same as that which it would exert if it alone occupied the container.
Alteration of the state of a gas without allowing the temperature to alter is known as adiabatic change.

1.78   **Answers: B C D**

The critical temperature is the temperature above which a substance cannot be liquefied by pressure alone. The critical temperature applies to a single gas. The pseudocritical temperature is the temperature at which gas mixtures separate out into their constituent parts.

1.79   **Answers: B E**

Absolute humidity is the amount of water vapour per unit volume of gas at a given temperature and pressure. In the upper trachea absolute humidity is 34 g/m³ or 34 mg/l. Humidification avoids the need for latent heat of vaporisation which normally accounts for 15% of total heat loss within the trachea. < 2% of basal heat loss is used to warm the gases. HMEs are now > 70% efficient and can give a humidity of the inspired gases of > 20 g/m³. Each HME should only be used for a maximum of 24 hours. There is a risk of increased airways resistance (i.e. increased work of breathing) due to dry crusted secretions and infection.

1.80   **Answers: A B C D**

Thermocouples rely on the Seebeck effect i.e. when two dissimilar conductors are joined together to form a circuit, a potential difference is generated, the size of which is proportional to the difference in temperatures of the two junctions. In order to measure temperature one junction has to be kept at a constant temperature. Alcohol thermometers are more suitable for measuring very low temperatures as mercury solidifies at –39°C. However, they are unsuitable for measuring high temperatures as alcohol boils at 78.5°C.

The resistance thermometer relies on the fact that the electrical resistance of a metal increases linearly with temperature. A thermistor also uses resistance to measure temperature. It consists of a bead of metal oxide, the resistance of which falls exponentially as temperature rises. The interferometer is used for gas analysis.

1.81   **Answers: A D**

The Wright's respirometer is a turbine flowmeter used to measure expiratory gas volumes. It gives falsely low readings when the ventilation volumes to be measured are small and when the vanes are wet. It over reads when flow rates or tidal volumes are great. It also gives slightly higher readings with mixtures of nitrous oxide and oxygen than for air. To improve accuracy, the respirometer should be positioned as close as possible to the patient's trachea on the expiratory limb of the breathing circuit. The Wright's respirometer is calibrated for use for tidal volume measurement and for tidal ventilation. Its calibration is inaccurate if it is used to measure a continuous flow.

1.82   **Answers: A C D**

Evoked potentials (EPs) are electrical potentials recorded from the central nervous system or peripherally following repetitive central or peripheral stimulation. EPs can be sensory (e.g. somatosensory, auditory or visual) or motor.

1.83   **Answers: C D**

The half-life is the time taken for the initial response to fall to half its value. As an alternative to half-life, the rate of an exponential process can be measured by its time constant. It is equal to the time at which the process would have been complete had the initial rate of change continued. After 1 time constant the process is 63% complete, after 2 time constants it is 86.5% complete, after 3 time constants it is 95% complete and after 4 time constants it is 99.75% complete.

1.84   **Answers: A C D E**

Resistance = driving pressure/gas flow rate. Driving pressure is the difference between alveolar and mouth pressures and can be measured with the body plethysmograph. Gas flow rate can be measured with a pneumotachograph. Airway resistance is the pressure difference between the alveoli and the mouth per unit of air flow. It is therefore measured in cmH_2O L s-π or kPa L s-π. Airway resistance increases during inhalational anaesthesia. This may be caused by the reduced functional residual capacity and lung volume or by the tubes and connections of the breathing system. PEEP reduces airway resistance according to the inverse relationship between lung volume and airway resistance; it recruits previously closed alveoli.

1.85   **Answers: A B C E**

Microshock refers to the application of a small current close to or directly to the heart. Cardiac pacing wires and invasive monitoring catheters provide a conductive route to the endothelium of the heart. Blood and saline can act as electrical conductors. Under these circumstances currents as low as 100 µA can result in ventricular fibrillation. Ideally two or more pieces of earthed equipment should be at the same potential to avoid leakage currents which can give rise to microelectrocution. However, it is virtually impossible to ensure that all earth connections which are made to the patient, either deliberately or accidentally are at the same potential. It is therefore recommended that patients are isolated from earth by using isolated or floating circuits.

1.86   **Answers: A C**

Refer to Answer 1.57.

1.87   **Answers: A B C D**

The Lack system is a coaxial modification of the Magill Mapleson A system. The Magill and Lack systems are efficient for spontaneous ventilation; fresh gas flow (FGF) required = alveolar minute ventilation (approximately 70 ml/kg). However, although they can be used for controlled ventilation, they are very inefficient; FGF required = 3 x alveolar minute ventilation.

1.88   **Answers: A B C D**

The central venous pressure (CVP) is expressed as cmH_2O or mmHg above a point level with the right atrium e.g. midaxillary line. When changing the position of the patient it is important that the pressure recorded always be related to the level of the right atrium.

Misplacement of the catheter may lead to inaccuracies e.g. if the catheter tip is in the right ventricle; this leads to an unexpectedly high pressure with pronounced oscillations. This is easily distinguished when the waveform is displayed. The upper end of the manometer column is open to air via a cotton wool filter. The filter must stay dry to maintain direct connection with the atmosphere. Straining causes a raised intrathoracic pressure, increasing CVP. Measurement of the CVP is useful in shock and hypovolaemia.

1.89   **Answers: A B C D E**

Static electricity and dirt on the bobbin can both cause the bobbin to stick. Dirt is a particular problem at low flow rates when the clearance between the bobbin and flowmeter wall is narrow. Each rotameter is calibrated for a specific gas at room temperature and pressure. Minute volume divider ventilators exert back pressure as they cycle. A flow restrictor can be fitted downstream of the flowmeters to prevent this from happening. As altitude increases barometric pressure decreases. At low flow rates, flow is laminar and dependent on gas viscosity, a property which is independent of altitude. At high flow rates, flow becomes turbulent and flow is dependent on density, a property which is influenced by altitude. The decrease in density at altitude increases the actual flow rate and so the flowmeter under reads.

1.90   **Answers: B E**

Capnography works on the absorption of carbon dioxide (CO_2) from the infra-red spectrum. Collision broadening is where the absorption of carbon dioxide is increased due to the presence of nitrous oxide. This occurs because carbon dioxide can transfer some of its absorbed infra-red energy to nitrous oxide molecules when they collide. This results in the CO_2 molecules being able to absorb more energy than would otherwise be the case. The absorption spectrum of the nitrous oxide is broadened and hence the term 'collision broadening'. The $PaCO_2/PeCO_2$ gradient in normal subjects is approximately 0.4–0.7 kPa. The difference increases in V/Q mismatch.

STATION 1.1

Answers and explanations

(a) This is a chest X-ray showing a large pneumothorax.

(b)
&
(c) The film is an AP film; the heart appears magnified in AP views as it lies further from the X-ray plate and thus the X-rays are dispersed over a wider area. It is thus not possible to comment on heart size in AP films.

(d) To decide whether a film is rotated or not one should look at the clavicles and their relationship to each other. The clavicles should be horizontal and of equal length; it is in fact rather difficult to comment on whether this film is rotated or not.

(e) Clinically a pneumothorax may be detected by hyper-resonance on percussion, reduced air entry and deviation of the trachea away from the side of the pneumothorax.

(f) A pneumothorax of this size can cause compression of the mediastinum and reduced venous return leading to a reduction in cardiac output and even cardiac arrest. It requires urgent decompression; initially with a large bore iv cannula in the second intercostal space in the midclavicular line followed by insertion of a chest drain with underwater seal.

STATION 1.2

Answers and explanations

(a) **True**   (b) **False**   (c) **True**   (d) **True**   (e) **True**

(f) **False**   (g) **True**   (h) **True**   (i) **False**

The ECG shows trifascicular block. There is first degree heart block (a prolonged PR interval; greater than 0.2 s). There is a right bundle branch block pattern and left axis deviation.

The rate is normal; it is about 80 beats per minute.

To work out the rate, assuming a regular rhythm, one divides the number of large squares between two R waves by 300. The explanation for this is as follows:

The ECG speed is 25 mm/s. i.e.   5 large squares. Thus in 1 minute there are 60 x 5 large squares = 300.

Thus the rate is derived by the R-R interval divided by 300.

The rhythm on this ECG is sinus.

The calibration is shown by the 1 cm tall square at the extreme right of the ECG. 1 mV = 1 cm

Trifascicular block is an indication for the insertion of a permanent pacemaker as complete heart block may supervene.

Anaesthesia should not be undertaken until a pacemaker has been inserted. If the surgery is urgent a temporary pacing wire must be inserted.

STATION 1.3

Answers and explanations

(a) The patient has disseminated intravascular coagulation (DIC). There is evidence of consumption of clotting factors, fibrinogen and platelets.

(b) The management of DIC is essentially to replace the missing clotting factors and platelets with FFP, cryoprecipitate and platelets.

(c) The blood gas sample shows a mainly metabolic acidosis, although there is also a small respiratory component.

(d) There is clearly respiratory failure.

(e) Despite an inspired oxygen concentration of 70%, the PaO_2 is only 9.6 kPa. This implies a large shunt as the ideal alveolar gas equation states that

$$PaO_2 = FiO_2 - PaCO_2/R$$

In other words the PaO_2 should be about 60 kPa.

(f) The patient is clearly very unwell and needs intensive care management to optimise his condition prior to and after surgery.

STATION 1.4

Answers and explanations

These blood tests reveal severe liver and renal dysfunction.
The urea and creatinine are elevated and there is associated acidosis and hyperkalaemia.
The raised AST and bilirubin and the hyponatraemia are due to the hepatic failure.

(a) Other tests which are necessary at this time are an ECG, clotting screen and full blood count, chest X-ray, arterial blood gas sample and ultrasound of the kidneys and ureters.

(b) The ECG may show signs of hyperkalaemia; in any event this will need treating.
The CXR may show pulmonary oedema.
The clotting will be abnormal and the platelets may be low.
The blood gas will confirm and quantify the metabolic acidosis.
The ultrasound is to exclude a treatable obstructive uropathy.

(d) Anaesthesia is clearly to be deferred in this patient!
The patient needs ITU care, dialysis or haemofiltration and referral to a hepatologist.

STATION 1.5

Answer and explanations

Ischaemic heart disease increases the morbidity and mortality in general surgical patients. It is therefore important to take a history to assess the severity of the problem, especially as in this instance the patient is undergoing elective surgery.

The history should assess the man's exercise tolerance and whether he gets anginal chest pains. If he does suffer with angina then one needs to establish its frequency, exacerbating and relieving factors. One should ask about any prior myocardial infarcts or hospital admissions with angina.
His smoking history, current drug therapy and previous anaesthetic history are all relevant.

STATION 1.6

Answers and explanations

(a) The X-ray is of the cervical spine and shows atlanto-axial instability. This is diagnosed when the distance between the posterior aspect of the anterior arch of the atlas and the anterior aspect of the odontoid process exceeds 3 mm in adults or 5 mm in children.
This is most often found in patients with rheumatoid arthritis, but may also be seen in Down's syndrome, ankylosing spondylitis, psoriatic arthropathy or systemic lupus erythematosus.

(b) The significance of this finding is that there is a risk of cervical cord damage when the neck is extended; as happens during laryngoscopy.
If intubation is essential then the patient should wear a cervical collar and neck extension limited to the minimum amount of time necessary.

STATION 1.7

Answers and explanations

(a) She should be prescribed ranitidine to reduce gastric acid production and metoclopramide to promote gastric emptying and increase lower oesophageal sphincter tone.
The aim is to reduce the volume and acidity of stomach contents and the likelihood of regurgitation, aspiration and pneumonitis. She should also be given sodium citrate prior to induction.

(b) A rapid sequence induction with cricoid pressure should be performed to minimise the risk of aspiration.

STATION 1.8

Answers and explanations

(a) The likelihood is that she has taken an overdose of salicylate (aspirin).
This would explain the symptoms and would be in keeping with the blood gas findings.

(b) Aspirin can lead to a range of metabolic disturbances.
Initially the salicylate stimulates the respiratory centre in the brain causing hyperventilation and leading to a respiratory alkalosis.
In more severe overdose there is a metabolic acidosis which is due to the acid load and because aspirin leads to the uncoupling of oxidative phosphorylation.
In many cases, as in this example, there is a mixed respiratory alkalosis and metabolic acidosis.
Sweating, hyperpyrexia, gastrointestinal bleeding and a coagulopathy may occur.

(c) Management may include gastric lavage, forced alkaline diuresis and haemodialysis.

STATION 1.9

Answer and explanation

Having introduced yourself to both mother and child you should then explain the options for analgesia.

The child should have EMLA cream although at this age a gaseous induction may be used as an alternative.

A general anaesthetic with either a caudal or penile block may be employed.

You should explain that both techniques are safe and effective. If, for instance, the mother has had an epidural for labour then the caudal might be explained as a mini epidural.

The use of rectal non-steroidal anti-inflammatory analgesics are, it should be explained, very safe, routine and effective.

However if the mother refuses any of the above forms of analgesia then her wishes must be respected.

STATION 1.10

Answers and explanation

(a) Basic Life Support (BLS) should be initiated:
First check for responsiveness by shaking the patient and shouting. In this case there is no response.

Shout for help, open his airway with head tilt and chin lift, removing any visible obstruction if present.

Check for breathing by looking, listening and feeling for 10 seconds only. In this case there is no breathing.

In the DIY store there will be other people around. Send one of them to telephone for an ambulance.

Give 2 rescue breaths and check the carotid pulse for 10 seconds.

If a pulse is present: continue rescue breathing until he starts breathing on his own. Check pulse (for 10 seconds only) every minute.

If no pulse is present: start chest compressions – depress sternum 4–5 cm at a rate of 100 per minute. Combine this with rescue breathing (with a ratio of 15 chest compressions to 2 breaths) unless there is someone in the store who is trained and proficient in BLS in which case 2 person BLS is the preferred method (with a ratio of 5 chest compressions to 1 breath)

Time should not be wasted by checking the pulse again unless the patient takes a spontaneous breath or moves.

Remember that if there is any suspicion of a spinal cord injury, jaw thrust should be used rather than head tilt and chin lift.

(b) The ECG shows ventricular fibrillation.

Defibrillation is the priority now. The chances of successful defibrillation decrease with time and diminish by 5–10% per minute, although this process is slowed down by BLS.

The initial 3 shocks are given at 200 J, 200 J and 360 J. The carotid pulse should only be palpated if after any of the shocks, the rhythm changes to one compatible with a cardiac output.

Subsequent shocks are given at 360 J unless a spontaneous cardiac output is restored during the resuscitation, which then reverts back to ventricular fibrillation or pulseless ventricular tachycardia, in which case the sequence is 200 J, 200 J and 360 J.

The airway can be secured with tracheal intubation and the patient ventilated with 100% oxygen. Intravenous access is gained and adrenaline 1 mg given every 3 minutes.

It is vital to transfer the patient to hospital for more advanced management e.g. lignocaine, bretylium, sodium bicarbonate, central venous access, etc.

In the out-of-hospital situation at least some of the potentially reversible causes of cardiac arrest can be ruled out/treated – hypoxia, hypovolaemia, tension pneumothorax.

STATION 1.11

Answers and explanation

Laminar flow through a cannula is directly proportional to the fourth power of the radius and inversely related to the length of the cannula. Thus the ideal is a short, wide-bore cannula. CVP catheters are long and not particularly wide-bore and are thus not the ideal for rapid fluid administration.

A 14 gauge Venflon approximates to the ideal and can deliver at maximal flow rate of 270 ml/min.

Flow is also inversely related to the viscosity of the fluid being administered; thus crystalloid and colloid can be given more rapidly than blood.

For very rapid fluid, particularly blood, administration a Swan Ganz sheath side port is particularly effective.

STATION 1.12

Answers and explanations

(a) The photograph shows a cylinder of Entonox.

(b) Entonox is a 50:50 mixture of oxygen and nitrous oxide.

(c) The critical temperature of nitrous oxide is 36.5°C; that of oxygen -118°C.

(d) When the two gases are mixed together, due to a phenomenon known as the Poynting effect, the pseudocritical temperature is -8°C.

(e) If a cylinder of Entonox cools to below its pseudocritical temperature the two gases separate out. The result is that initially the patient receives almost pure oxygen and therefore no analgesia and then, once the oxygen is used up, pure nitrous oxide; a potentially lethal hypoxic mixture.

STATION 1.13

Answers and explanation

The patient needs to lie supine and head down about 15 degrees.
The head down tilt engorges the internal jugular vein thus making it easier to access and also reduces the risk of air embolism.
The operator needs to wash, gown and glove; the technique must be strictly aseptic. The patient's neck should be prepared with a cleaning antiseptic lotion and towels put over the area.
The approach to the vein is located by finding the apex of a triangle formed by the two heads of sternocleidomastoid and the clavicle.
The needle is angulated at 45 degrees to the horizontal, aiming for the ipsilateral nipple. The vein is often very superficial, no more than a centimetre or two beneath the skin.
Once the vein is entered a Seldinger wire is passed through the needle. The needle is withdrawn and the plastic catheter passed over the wire; the wire is then itself withdrawn. The catheter is sewn in place and a dressing put over it.

(a) The incidence of pneumothorax is far less via the internal jugular route compared with the subclavian.

(b) There are many possible complications, apart from failure to cannulate the vein. Amongst the most common are accidental arterial puncture, pneumothorax and air embolism. Infection at the site is a potential late complication.

STATION 1.14

Answers and explanation

(a) Other rare causes of convulsions include herpes simplex encephalitis and biochemical disturbances such as hypoglycaemia or hyponatraemia.

(b) There is significant morbidity associated with eclamptic convulsions. The initial management of the situation is to maintain an airway, ensure adequate ventilation and to terminate the seizures.
Intravenous Diazemuls, followed with a loading dose of magnesium is the way to terminate the seizures. To prevent further convulsions a magnesium infusion should be commenced. The magnesium levels must be measured and the patient clinically examined for signs of magnesium toxicity. Intravenous calcium gluconate is the

antidote for magnesium toxicity.

Once the situation is stabilised the baby should be delivered by caesarean section.

STATION 1.15

Answers and explanation

(a) This is the normal/Gaussian distribution curve.
(b) It represents continuous data.
(c) The mean, median and mode are represented by the same point.
     Pain scores are an example of ordinal data i.e. non-parametric data.
(d) Student's t-test is used for parametric data.

STATION 1.16

Answer

Cricoid pressure is a manoeuvre that is used either to facilitate intubation or as part of a rapid sequence induction to prevent aspiration of acidic gastric contents.

To perform cricoid pressure the operator presses down on the cricoid cartilage. The cricoid is located immediately below the Adam's apple, the thyroid cartilage.

The operator should apply 44 Newtons pressure; approximately the pressure needed to register 3.5 kg on a set of weighing scales!

The cricoid cartilage compresses the oesophagus between it and the body of the 6th cervical vertebra, thus preventing the passage of any regurgitated gastric contents beyond this point.

The patient should be warned prior to performing the manoeuvre; it should be applied in the context of a rapid sequence induction immediately prior to administering the induction agent.

If a patient actively vomits whilst cricoid pressure is being applied the pressure must be released as there may otherwise be a danger of oesophageal rupture.

Viva 1a

PHARMACOLOGY
Muscle relaxants

What types of muscle relaxants do you know?
There are two types of muscle relaxant; depolarising and non-depolarising.

What are the differences between the two groups?
Depolarising muscle relaxants
- Muscle fasciculations occur before the onset of neuromuscular blockade
- Show equal but diminished responses to train of four or tetanic stimulation
- Progression to dual block can occur
- Anticholinesterases potentiate the neuromuscular blockade

Non-depolarising muscle relaxants
- No muscle fasciculations
- Display 'fade' with train of four or tetanic stimulation
- Post-tetanic facilitation occurs i.e. there is an increased twitch height following tetanic stimulation
- Anticholinesterases reverse the block produced by these agents

How does a depolarising muscle relaxant work? Name two.
Depolarising agents resemble acetylcholine structurally and act by mimicking acetylcholine. They bind to the acetylcholine receptors where they elicit opening of the sodium channels and muscle depolarisation (causing the characteristic muscle fasciculations). However, this receptor activation is prolonged as they do not dissociate from the acetylcholine receptor as rapidly as acetylcholine and a sustained receptor activation results. Persistent endplate depolarisation causes inactivation of the voltage-sensitive sodium channels and muscle relaxation.
Suxamethonium and decamethonium are depolarising muscle relaxants.

What is the principle behind the speed of onset of non-depolarising muscle relaxants?
Studies have suggested that rapid onset of a non-depolarising block can only occur by giving large doses of the non-depolarising agent. This has important implications in that, if a large dose of a relatively potent drug is given, a fast speed of onset will occur but there will be a prolonged blockade time.

What can you tell me about rocuronium?
Rocuronium bromide is a relatively new non-depolarising neuromuscular blocker with an amino-steroid structure similar to vecuronium. It comes in a 10 mg/ml solution for intravenous use.
As with other non-depolarising agents, it acts by competing with acetylcholine for its receptor but is unable to induce the conformational changes necessary at the nicotinic acetylcholine receptor for ion channel opening and subsequent depolarisation of the postsynaptic membrane. The intubating dose of rocuronium is 0.6 mg/kg. It is eliminated in bile and urine 70% unchanged, 3-hydroxyrocuronium being the only known metabolite. Its advantages over other muscle relaxants are: very fast onset (almost as fast as suxamethonium without all its side-effects) with good intubating conditions in 60–90 seconds and yet a duration of action similar to vecuronium and atracurium. This is thought to be due to its low potency. Virtually free of cardiovascular effects and no significant histamine release.

PHYSIOLOGY
Inotropes

What is an inotrope?
An inotrope is a drug which increases myocardial contractility.

Classify inotropes.
Catecholamines
- Increase cAMP and intracellular calcium concentrations
- May be naturally occurring or synthetic
  Adrenaline - α and β agonist
  Noradrenaline - mainly α, some β
  Isoprenaline - β agonist only
  Dopamine - α, β and D1 agonist
  Dobutamine - mainly β_1 agonist, weak α and β_2 effect
  Dopexamine - β_2, D1 and D2 agonist

Phosphodiesterase inhibitors
- Increase cAMP concentrations by preventing its breakdown
- Positive inotropism and vasodilatation (inodilators)
- Little effect on myocardial oxygen demand
  Specific – enoximone, amrinone, milrinone
  Non-specific – aminophylline

Cardiac glycosides
- Inhibit the action of the $Na^+/K^+ATPase$ in cell membranes, increasing intracellular Na^+ which displaces bound intracellular calcium ions

Calcium
- Has a transient positive inotropic effect by increasing intracellular calcium ions

Glucagon
- Causes increased cAMP concentrations and intracellular calcium release by acting on an unknown receptor

Discuss Dopexamine.
Dopexamine is a synthetic catecholamine, presented as 10 mg/ml (1%) dopexamine hydrochloride for intravenous administration. β_2, D1 and D2 agonist, increases cardiac output without significantly changing myocardial oxygen consumption. Its actions are arterial vasodilatation including renal and splanchnic vessels, weak positive inotrope (-β_2 and inhibition of uptake 1). The dosage is 0.5–6 µg/kg/min and duration of action is $t^{1/2}$ = 5–10 mins. Extensively metabolised in the liver and excreted in bile and urine. The side-effects include: arrhythmias, angina, tremor, flushing, headache, nausea and vomiting.

Viva 1b

CLINICAL

How would you anaesthetise her?
I would first ask for senior assistance as she is a high risk case.
She needs to be fully fluid resuscitated, preferably on an intensive care unit with central venous pressure guidance.
An arterial line, urinary catheter and nasogastric tube should all be inserted.

Before her anaesthetic her confusion should be further investigated in view of her previous history of cerebrovascular accidents.

Once deemed fit for anaesthesia she should be pre-oxygenated with full monitoring in place. A rapid sequence induction should be carried out.

What are the options for post-operative analgesia?
In view of her abnormal clotting profile an epidural is contraindicated.

Non-steroidal anti-inflammatory drugs should be avoided in view of her renal impairment.

Opiates and simple analgesics such as paracetamol remain the only options.

In view of her confusion a patient controlled analgesia (PCA) pump is unlikely to be practicable and therefore intermittent intramuscular morphine seems the most applicable solution.

PHYSICS
Compare laminar and turbulent flow.

Laminar flow
- Smooth orderly flow in a straight line in one direction
- Fluid flows parallel to the vessel wall
- Velocity is highest in the centre of the vessel, decreasing towards the periphery and approaching zero at the wall (parabolic velocity profile)
- The type of flow seen in smooth tubes at low flows
- Affected by viscosity

Turbulent flow
- Flow is less organised with eddy currents causing fluid flow in all directions although there is a general progression along the tube
- Occurs at high flow rates, sharp angles, branching points and where there are changes in diameter or irregularities in the tube
- Affected by changes in density
- Compared with laminar flow, a greater pressure difference is required to maintain the same flow rate (i.e. there is a greater resistance to flow)

Do you have any equations explaining these? What is the Reynolds' number?
Laminar flow through a tube is described by the Hageni-Poiseuille equation : $V = \Delta P \pi r^4 / 8 \eta \lambda$ where V = rate of flow, ΔP = pressure gradient along tube, r = radius of tube, η = viscosity of fluid and l = length of tube.
For turbulent flow: flow rate is proportional to $\Delta P (r2)/\Delta \rho$ where ΔP = pressure gradient along tube, r = radius of tube and ρ = density of fluid.

Reynold's number = vpd/η where v = linear velocity, p = gas density, d = diameter of tube and η = gas viscosity. Reynold's number is used to predict whether flow is laminar or turbulent. If it is greater than 2000, turbulent flow is likely. A value less than 1000 is associated with laminar flow. Between 1000 and 2000 both types of flow occur.

Are there any pieces of equipment based on the principle of laminar flow?
The pneumotachograph is based on the principle of laminar flow.

Explain how a pneumotachograph works.
A pneumotachograph is a constant orifice variable pressure instrument used to measure gas flow rate. It does this by measuring the pressure drop across a laminar resistance.

PRACTICE EXAMINATION 2

90 Questions: time allowed 3 hours.
Indicate your answers with a tick or cross in the spaces provided.

2.1   Recognised complications of dextran infusions are

- ❏ A   antigenic reactions
- ❏ B   problems with cross matching of blood
- ❏ C   an increase in venous thrombosis
- ❏ D   renal failure
- ❏ E   an increase in rouleaux formation

2.2   The level of serum potassium may be

- ❏ A   increased by suxamethonium
- ❏ B   increased by thiopentone
- ❏ C   increased by metabolic alkalosis
- ❏ D   affected by extensive burns
- ❏ E   reduced by D-tubocurarine

2.3   Non-depolarising muscle relaxants

- ❏ A   produce post tetanic facilitation
- ❏ B   all have their action prolonged by alkalosis
- ❏ C   produce fasciculation
- ❏ D   can exhibit dual block
- ❏ E   have a prolonged action in severe hypothermia

2.4   Convulsions occurring intra-operatively or in the early post-operative period may be due to

- ❏ A   ether
- ❏ B   suxamethonium
- ❏ C   halothane
- ❏ D   bupivacaine
- ❏ E   hypoxia

2.5 **After intravenous thiopentone, the following may occur:**

❑ A severe hypotension
❑ B respiratory depression
❑ C liver toxicity
❑ D pain at the injection site
❑ E epileptic convulsions

2.6 **At equivalent minimum alveolar concentration (MAC), comparing halothane with enflurane**

❑ A enflurane causes more respiratory depression than halothane
❑ B enflurane causes more cardiac arrhythmias than halothane
❑ C enflurane causes a greater fall in cardiac output than halothane
❑ D both release inorganic fluoride ions
❑ E enflurane has a higher boiling point than halothane

2.7 **Digoxin is indicated in**

❑ A atrial flutter
❑ B 2:1 block
❑ C ventricular tachycardia
❑ D nodal tachycardia
❑ E Stokes-Adams attacks

2.8 **Propranolol is contraindicated in**

❑ A bronchial asthma
❑ B the presence of a low serum potassium
❑ C paroxysmal nocturnal dyspnoea
❑ D patients already on digoxin
❑ E atrial fibrillation

2.9 **Dopamine infused at a dosage of 10 µg/kg/min would produce**

❏ A increased urinary output
❏ B increased sodium output
❏ C increased cardiac output
❏ D multiple ventricular extrasystoles
❏ E an unchanged peripheral resistance

2.10 **Ketamine**

❏ A raises intracranial pressure
❏ B causes muscle relaxation
❏ C relaxes the uterus
❏ D is excreted in the urine
❏ E premedication with atropine is advisable when it is used

2.11 **Sodium dantrolene**

❏ A is a neuromuscular blocker
❏ B may cause a dangerous rise in the serum calcium
❏ C can be used pre-operatively to reduce suxamethonium pains
❏ D is useful in the treatment of malignant hyperpyrexia
❏ E is a skeletal muscle relaxant

2.12 **Isoflurane**

❏ A has the same molecular weight as enflurane
❏ B if put in a calibrated halothane vaporiser (i.e. Fluotec), will deliver a dangerously high concentration of isoflurane
❏ C reduces the blood pressure, mainly by depressing cardiac output
❏ D has a MAC of 1.68%
❏ E causes minimal changes in cerebral blood flow at light levels of anaesthesia

2.13 Morphine

- ❏ A may cause histamine release
- ❏ B decreases catecholamine levels
- ❏ C causes miosis
- ❏ D causes vomiting by direct stimulation of the vomiting centre
- ❏ E arterial pCO_2 is markedly raised with normal therapeutic dosage

2.14 Chlorpromazine

- ❏ A is a weak antihistamine
- ❏ B is an alpha blocker
- ❏ C can cause Parkinsonism
- ❏ D is an anti-emetic
- ❏ E has an atropine like action

2.15 Chlorpropamide

- ❏ A has a half-life of 12 hours
- ❏ B is mainly metabolised in the liver
- ❏ C causes alcohol intolerance in about 30% of patients
- ❏ D acts by stimulating insulin production
- ❏ E results in unwanted effects twice as commonly as tolbutamide

2.16 The MAC value of an inhalational anaesthetic agent will be influenced by

- ❏ A the age of the patient
- ❏ B the concomitant administration of morphine
- ❏ C a change in the arterial pCO_2 from 3.5 to 6.5 kPa
- ❏ D its blood/gas partition coefficient
- ❏ E the use of nitrous oxide with it

2.17 Halothane decreases the blood pressure as a result of

- ❏ A direct myocardial depression
- ❏ B peripheral vasodilatation
- ❏ C a central action on the vasomotor centre
- ❏ D ganglion blockade
- ❏ E baroreceptor inhibition

2.18 Bupivacaine

- ❏ A produces depolarisation in the neural membrane of peripheral nerves
- ❏ B is detoxified in the liver
- ❏ C is an ester
- ❏ D can cause methaemoglobinaemia
- ❏ E 30 ml of 0.5% is the recommended dose in a 75 kg man

2.19 The following are anticonvulsant:

- ❏ A diazepam
- ❏ B chlormethiazole
- ❏ C oxazepam
- ❏ D chlorpropamide
- ❏ E thiopentone

2.20 Albumin

- ❏ A has a molecule weight of approximately 65,000 Daltons
- ❏ B is increased in chronic liver disease
- ❏ C is increased in malabsorption syndrome
- ❏ D makes a significant contribution to plasma oncotic pressure
- ❏ E has a normal value of 34–45 g/l

2.21   The following cause methaemoglobinaemia:

❑ A   atropine
❑ B   prilocaine
❑ C   methylene blue
❑ D   cyanide
❑ E   higher oxides of nitrogen

2.22   The following are anti-emetics:

❑ A   hyoscine
❑ B   carbimazole
❑ C   perphenazine
❑ D   apomorphine
❑ E   cyclizine

2.23   Thiazide diuretics

❑ A   act on the proximal convoluted tubule
❑ B   cause hyponatraemia
❑ C   increase serum uric acid
❑ D   cause hypercalcaemia
❑ E   potentiate digoxin

2.24   Ketamine causes

❑ A   bradycardia
❑ B   postural hypotension
❑ C   increased intracranial pressure
❑ D   delirium
❑ E   muscle rigidity

2.25 The following potentiate a competitive neuromuscular block:

❑ A magnesium
❑ B calcium
❑ C increased or decreased potassium
❑ D hyperventilation
❑ E increased or decreased pH

2.26 Sodium nitroprusside cyanide toxicity is

❑ A due to free cyanide
❑ B due to thiocyanate
❑ C worse in the presence of vitamin B12 deficiency
❑ D worse in liver rhodanese deficiency
❑ E dose-dependent

2.27 Propranolol

❑ A can cause hypoglycaemia
❑ B causes bradycardia
❑ C is a bronchoconstrictor
❑ D acts via cyclic AMP
❑ E is potentiated by enoximone

2.28 Frusemide

❑ A can cause a reduction in blood sugar
❑ B decreases blood volume
❑ C reduces osmolality in the renal tubules
❑ D acts in the proximal convoluted tubule
❑ E causes hyperkalaemia

2.29 Ventricular tachycardia can be abolished by

- ❏ A digoxin
- ❏ B lignocaine
- ❏ C verapamil
- ❏ D disopyramide
- ❏ E adenosine

2.30 The speed of induction of an inhalational agent is increased by

- ❏ A hypovolaemia
- ❏ B hyperventilation
- ❏ C increased cardiac output
- ❏ D high solubility of the agent
- ❏ E polycythaemia

2.31 Long-term deficiency of adrenal cortical hormones causes

- ❏ A hyperpigmentation
- ❏ B hypovolaemia
- ❏ C hyponatraemia
- ❏ D hypokalaemia
- ❏ E decrease in anterior pituitary functions

2.32 Angiotensin II

- ❏ A stimulates the thirst centre
- ❏ B causes marked arteriolar vasoconstriction
- ❏ C causes venoconstriction
- ❏ D causes release of aldosterone from the zona glomerulosa
- ❏ E is metabolised in the lungs

2.33 Gastrin is

- ❑ A released in response to acid in the antrum
- ❑ B released in response to ethanol in the antrum
- ❑ C released from the fundus
- ❑ D increased by acetylcholine
- ❑ E increased by sympathetic stimulation

2.34 Clearance

- ❑ A equals renal excretion divided by plasma concentration
- ❑ B of urea equals glomerular filtration rate (GFR)
- ❑ C of PAH equals renal plasma blood flow
- ❑ D of inulin is less than that of glucose
- ❑ E of free water is greater than that of inulin

2.35 Physiological dead space

- ❑ A changes with posture
- ❑ B decreases with exercise
- ❑ C includes anatomical dead space
- ❑ D is responsible for the difference between mixed expired gas and alveolar gas
- ❑ E is diffusion dependent

2.36 Lung surfactant

- ❑ A decreases compliance
- ❑ B increases surface tension
- ❑ C is released from the pulmonary circulation
- ❑ D is made of molecules that are partly lipophilic and partly hydrophilic
- ❑ E is produced in type I pneumocytes

2.37   The pyramidal tract

❏   A   is named after the cells in the cortex where it originates
❏   B   has 1 million fibres, 80–90% of which decussate in the medulla
❏   C   comes from area IV of the cortex
❏   D   is concerned with fine movements
❏   E   will degenerate after decortication

2.38   Smooth, cardiac and skeletal muscle have the following in common:

❏   A   gap junctions where electrical transmission spreads from cell to cell
❏   B   resting membrane potential
❏   C   action potential duration 200 ms
❏   D   all calcium ions for contraction come from intracellular storage
❏   E   contraction depends on interaction between actin and myosin

2.39   The pulmonary circulation

❏   A   contains 30% of the blood volume
❏   B   pulmonary vascular resistance increases with hypoxia
❏   C   pulmonary vascular resistance is markedly less than systemic vascular resistance
❏   D   pulmonary artery pressure is 25/9 mm Hg
❏   E   pulmonary artery pressure increases with exercise

2.40   At birth

❏   A   the ductus arteriosus opens
❏   B   left atrial pressure decreases
❏   C   pulmonary vascular resistance increases
❏   D   intrapleural pressure rises
❏   E   fetal haemoglobin is immediately replaced by HbA

2.41   Carbon dioxide

❏ A   is mainly carried as carbamino compounds
❏ B   10–15% is dissolved in the plasma
❏ C   crosses the placenta more easily than oxygen
❏ D   in fetal haemoglobin, carriage is facilitated by deoxygenation
❏ E   is more soluble in blood than oxygen

2.42   In a fit young person, tachycardia will be seen with

❏ A   emotional syncope
❏ B   expiration
❏ C   decrease in blood pressure
❏ D   noradrenaline infusion
❏ E   increased circulating thyroxine

2.43   Hypoxaemia stimulates ventilation by an effect on

❏ A   the carotid body
❏ B   the carotid sinus
❏ C   central chemoreceptors in the medulla
❏ D   central respiratory neurones
❏ E   cortical cells

2.44   Concerning skeletal muscle

❏ A   each fibre has one motor endplate
❏ B   the motor endplate is at the proximal end of the fibre
❏ C   depolarisation causes electrical changes only in the muscle
        fibre near the endplate
❏ D   the resting potential difference at the endplate is 20 mV less
        than the rest of the muscle
❏ E   each fibre is no longer than 1 mm

2.45   Section of the dorsal root nerves C3–L2 causes

☐   A   hypotonia
☐   B   paralysis
☐   C   loss of reflexes
☐   D   loss of sensation
☐   E   loss of supply to sympathetic sweat glands

2.46   In normal blood

☐   A   20 ml of oxygen is carried per 100 ml of plasma
☐   B   oxygen combines with globin in haemoglobin
☐   C   viscosity is largely due to red cells
☐   D   as velocity increases, red cells accumulate in the centre of vessels
☐   E   red cells metabolise glucose

2.47   Receptors in the carotid body

☐   A   respond to increases in $PaCO_2$ by increasing ventilation
☐   B   respond to stagnant hypoxia
☐   C   respond to haemorrhagic hypoxia
☐   D   have the same blood flow (weight for weight) as the myocardium
☐   E   do not respond to increasing pH by increasing ventilation

2.48   Valsalva manoeuvre is associated with

☐   A   increased central venous pressure
☐   B   decreased peripheral resistance
☐   C   tachycardia
☐   D   drop in blood pressure
☐   E   increased blood volume in the pulmonary circulation

2.49   The cerebrospinal fluid

❏   A   contains virtually no glucose
❏   B   pH does not accurately reflect the plasma pH
❏   C   is secreted by the choroid plexus
❏   D   is reabsorbed by the arachnoid villi
❏   E   pressure increases with compression of jugular veins

2.50   Agglutination will occur if the following donor blood is given to the following recipients:

		Donor	Recipient
❏	A	Group O	Group AB
❏	B	Group A	Group O
❏	C	Group AB	Group A
❏	D	Group A	Group AB
❏	E	Group O	Group A

2.51   Concerning the transmitter at motor nerve terminals

❏   A   it is formed from choline and acetyl coenzyme A
❏   B   formation occurs in the cleft
❏   C   it is broken down by pseudocholinesterase
❏   D   it has a muscarinic action
❏   E   release is increased by botulinum toxin

2.52   Enkephalin

❏   A   is a pentapeptide
❏   B   is the same as endorphin
❏   C   has a long half-life in the brain
❏   D   is mainly found in the pituitary
❏   E   is an agonist at opiate receptors but is not antagonised by naloxone

2.53   The following are beta actions of adrenaline:

☐   A   pupil dilation
☐   B   fine tremor
☐   C   tachycardia
☐   D   increase in cyclic AMP
☐   E   vasoconstriction

2.54   The following are effects of cortisol:

☐   A   protein anabolism
☐   B   osteoporosis
☐   C   potassium retention
☐   D   depression of function of the anterior pituitary
☐   E   salt and water retention

2.55   The plasma osmolality decreases after infusion of

☐   A   isotonic saline solution
☐   B   vasopressin
☐   C   aldosterone
☐   D   isotonic glucose
☐   E   20% albumin solution

2.56   Thyroid stimulating hormone (TSH) produces

☐   A   increased thyroidal uptake of iodine
☐   B   increased coupling of monoiodotyrosine and diiodotyrosine
☐   C   increased synthesis of thyroglobulin
☐   D   increased cyclic AMP levels in thyroid cells
☐   E   an increase in basal metabolic rate

2.57 **Which of the following are not seen following total pancreatectomy?**

❏ A little change in plasma insulin level
❏ B little change in plasma glucagon level
❏ C steatorrhoea
❏ D increased plasma levels of free fatty acids
❏ E decreased plasma $PaCO_2$

2.58 **Large doses of glucagon**

❏ A increase the force of contraction of the myocardium
❏ B increase the concentration of amino acids in the plasma
❏ C increase the concentration of free fatty acids in the plasma
❏ D decrease the plasma sodium concentration
❏ E stimulate the sympathetic nervous system

2.59 **A decreased extracellular fluid volume would be expected to cause an increased secretion of**

❏ A vasopressin
❏ B renin
❏ C ACTH
❏ D thyroxine
❏ E progesterone

2.60 **A high plasma calcium level causes**

❏ A bone demineralisation
❏ B decreased secretion of calcitonin
❏ C increased formation of 1,25 dihydroxycholecalciferol
❏ D decreased blood coagulability
❏ E increased formation of 24,25 dihydroxycholecalciferol

2.61 **A Wright's respirometer will give a reading that is lower than the actual value where there is**

❑ A low flow of gas
❑ B 30% oxygen in the gas
❑ C nitrous oxide present
❑ D humidity in the respirometer
❑ E an intermittent flow of gas

2.62 **Evoked potential techniques for measuring depth of anaesthesia utilise the following stimuli:**

❑ A auditory
❑ B oesophageal contractions
❑ C somatosensory
❑ D visual
❑ E magnetic resonance

2.63 **Blood pressure measurements read 'high' when**

❑ A there is a narrow cuff
❑ B the cuff is deflated slowly
❑ C the arm is held horizontal when the patient is sitting upright
❑ D the arm is obese
❑ E the arm muscles are held tight

2.64 **Helium is used by divers because it**

❑ A has a low viscosity
❑ B has no narcotic effect
❑ C diffuses easily through the nose
❑ D is more dense than air
❑ E can be liquefied

2.65 **The chances of microshock occurring increases due to**

❑ A saline filled catheters
❑ B earth loop
❑ C multiple earth connections
❑ D isolated circuit
❑ E oesophageal electrocardiogram

2.66 **The following are required to measure the cardiac output by the Fick principle:**

❑ A arterial oxygen content
❑ B venous oxygen content
❑ C oxygen uptake
❑ D respiratory quotient
❑ E arterial carbon monoxide content

2.67 **The following data apply to medical gases:**

❑ A the pressures swing absorber oxygen concentrator delivers about 5% argon
❑ B nitrogen is a constituent of nitrous oxide in the concentration of 0.5%
❑ C helium is obtained by fractional distillation of atmospheric air
❑ D the main source of carbon dioxide gas is as the by-product of petroleum hydrocarbon reformation
❑ E nitrous oxide is manufactured by thermal decomposition of ammonium nitrate

2.68 **In exponential change**

❑ A the time constant is the time taken for the initial response to fall to half its value
❑ B in one time constant, 37% change is complete
❑ C in three time constants, 95% change is complete
❑ D the rate of change of a variable is proportional to the magnitude of the variable
❑ E the half-life is half the time constant

2.69   Airway resistance

❏   A   can be measured by plethysmography
❏   B   is measured in kPa per litre
❏   C   increases during inhalational anaesthesia
❏   D   increases at high inspiratory flow rates
❏   E   decreases with the application of positive end expiratory
          pressure

2.70   The single breath nitrogen test measures

❏   A   anatomical dead space
❏   B   physiological dead space
❏   C   distribution of gases
❏   D   diffusing capacity
❏   E   closing volume

2.71   The alveolar to arterial oxygen tension is increased from normal

❏   A   with high inspired oxygen
❏   B   during nitrous oxide uptake
❏   C   in Fallot's tetralogy
❏   D   with a decrease in functional residual capacity
❏   E   in the elderly

2.72   With medical oxygen

❏   A   the critical temperature is 36.5°C
❏   B   manufacture is by the fractional distillation of air
❏   C   explosions can occur if, under pressure, it comes into contact
          with oil or grease
❏   D   convulsions can be caused if it is given under hyperbaric
          conditions
❏   E   bone marrow depression can occur with prolonged
          administration

2.73 In nitrous oxide cylinders for medical use

- ❏ A the cylinder is initially full of liquid
- ❏ B nitrous oxide is produced by heating ammonium nitrate
- ❏ C contaminants may be tested for with moistened starch-iodide paper
- ❏ D the pressure gauge is proportional to the amount of nitrous oxide in the cylinder
- ❏ E contamination with nitric oxide may occur

2.74 Soda lime

- ❏ A is mainly calcium carbonate
- ❏ B can be used to scavenge nitrous oxide
- ❏ C needs water to absorb carbon dioxide
- ❏ D in a properly packed canister, half the volume should be space between the granules
- ❏ E gets hot in use

2.75 The Magill circuit

- ❏ A is an example of a Mapleson A circuit
- ❏ B is functionally similar to the Lack circuit
- ❏ C is suitable for children over 25 kg
- ❏ D is efficient during IPPV
- ❏ E during spontaneous ventilation rebreathing and hypercarbia will occur if the fresh gas flow is less than the minute volume

2.76 Inaccuracies in the measurement of central venous pressure may arise from

- ❏ A a change in the position of the patient
- ❏ B misplacement of the catheter
- ❏ C wetting of the cotton wool plug in the top of the manometer tube
- ❏ D straining during respiration
- ❏ E arterial hypotension

2.77   The accuracy of a rotameter may be affected by

❑   A   dirt on the bobbin
❑   B   static electricity
❑   C   passing the wrong gas through it
❑   D   back pressure from the Manley ventilator
❑   E   using it at high altitude

2.78   The critical temperature is

❑   A   the temperature at which a gas becomes liquid if the pressure is raised
❑   B   the temperature above which a gas cannot be liquefied by increasing pressure alone
❑   C   the temperature at which latent heat of vaporisation equals zero
❑   D   the temperature that separates gases from vapours
❑   E   always lower than the boiling point of the same gas

2.79   A new anaesthetic agent has a saturated vapour pressure at 20°C of 152 mmHg. If there is a total fresh gas flow of 4 l/min, of which 80 ml is diverted through the vaporiser, the inspired concentration will be approximately

❑   A   1.6%
❑   B   0.8%
❑   C   2%
❑   D   0.4%
❑   E   5%

2.80   The critical pressure is

❑   A   the maximum pressure to which a cylinder can be filled
❑   B   the pressure above which a liquid cannot evaporate
❑   C   the pressure at which vapour is in equilibrium with its liquid
❑   D   120 bar
❑   E   the pressure at which a gas ignites

2.81   The following are true for gases in cylinders:

❑   A   oxygen is stored at 150 bar
❑   B   nitrous oxide is stored at 137 bar
❑   C   nitrous oxide should contain 1% water vapour
❑   D   nitrous oxide should not be stored below –8°C
❑   E   size E cylinders of oxygen and nitrous oxide are generally used on a Boyle's machine

2.82   For laminar flow in a tube, the flow rate is directionally proportional to

❑   A   its length
❑   B   the fourth power of its radius
❑   C   the density of the gas or liquid flowing through it
❑   D   the pressure drop across it
❑   E   the viscosity of the gas or liquid flowing through it

2.83   The vapour pressure of a liquid

❑   A   is linearly related to temperature
❑   B   can exceed the normal atmospheric pressure
❑   C   is a function of barometric pressure
❑   D   maintains a constant percentage of the vapour in the gas phase in a closed space above the liquid irrespective of the total pressure
❑   E   determines the gram molecular volume of the vapour

2.84   Concerning fires and explosions in theatre

❑   A   the relative humidity in the theatre should be kept at about 55%
❑   B   air is safer than oxygen
❑   C   switches within the zone of risk should be spark proof
❑   D   the floor should be terrazzo on a well-conducting screed
❑   E   cotton fabrics are better than silk

2.85   Regarding the gas laws

❏ A   Boyle's law states that at a constant temperature, the volume of a given mass of gas varies directly with pressure
❏ B   Charles' law states that at a constant pressure, the volume of a given mass of gas varies directly with temperature
❏ C   state that at a constant volume, the absolute pressure of a given mass of gas varies indirectly with temperature
❏ D   enable the pressure gauge to act as a contents gauge on the nitrous oxide cylinder
❏ E   in a mixture of gases, the pressure exerted by each of the gases is the same as it would exert if it alone occupied the cylinder

2.86   Regarding heat loss

❏ A   respiration accounts for 20% of heat loss
❏ B   radiation accounts for 40% of heat loss
❏ C   conduction accounts for 30% of heat loss
❏ D   more heat is lost humidifying than warming inspired gases
❏ E   the fall in temperature in the first hour of anaesthesia is 0.7°C if the theatre temperature is 21–24°C

2.87   Capnography

❏ A   works on the absorption of carbon dioxide in the ultraviolet region of the spectrum
❏ B   if used in combination with pulse oximetry, it would reduce anaesthetic mishaps by 90%
❏ C   the $PaCO_2/PeCO_2$ gradient in a patient with V/Q mismatch is 0.7 kPa
❏ D   collision broadening may occur in the presence of oxygen
❏ E   there are two sampling methods: side and main stream

2.88 When using diathermy

❑ A a low frequency current is used to maximise safety
❑ B the degree of burning depends on the current density
❑ C the likelihood of the patient sustaining a burn is reduced by using a large neutral plate
❑ D the spark gap determines whether the diathermy is used in the cutting or coagulation mode
❑ E if the neutral plate is disconnected, the patient may sustain a burn under the ECG electrodes

2.89 Regarding flow in a cylinder

❑ A if it is laminar, the flow will be directly proportional to the viscosity of the fluid
❑ B if it is turbulent, the flow will be indirectly proportional to the viscosity of the fluid
❑ C if the Reynold's number is less than 2000, laminar flow is likely
❑ D if it is laminar, halving the diameter of the tube will reduce the flow by one eighth
❑ E if it is turbulent, the flow will be directly proportional to the pressure across the tube

2.90 When using invasive blood pressure monitoring

❑ A damping may be caused by clot formation in the cannula
❑ B the resonant frequency may be increased by decreasing the compliance of the tubing
❑ C the resonant frequency may be increased by increasing the width of the tubing
❑ D if under damped, the systolic and diastolic pressure will be overestimated
❑ E the flow in the flushing system should exceed 4 ml/hr so as to prevent clot formation

16 Stations: time allowed approximately 2 hours.

STATION 2.1

A young asthmatic patient presents with a cough.

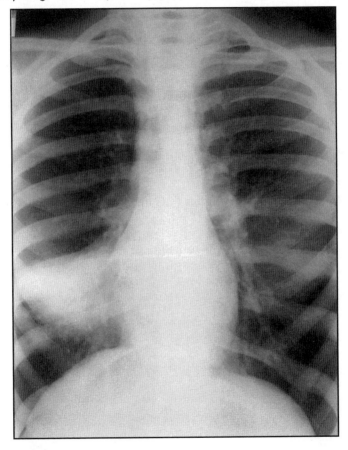

Fig. 2.1

What is the cause of this abnormal chest radiograph?

STATION 2.2

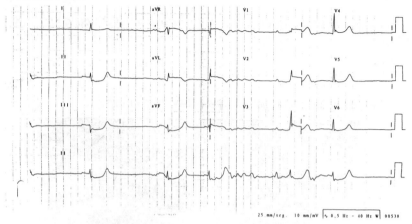

Fig. 2.2

(a) What is the diagnosis of this ECG?

(b) What are the features on this ECG that lead you to this diagnosis?

(c) How would you treat this patient?

STATION 2.3

Arterial blood gas analysis
pH 7.27   PaCO$_2$ 9.11   PaO$_2$ 7.93
HCO$_3$ 32   BE 8.5

(a) What picture is seen on the arterial blood gas analysis?

(b) Does this reflect an acute or chronic situation?

(c) Why is the HCO$_3$ high despite the low pH?

(d) What is the medical management of this patient?

STATION 2.4

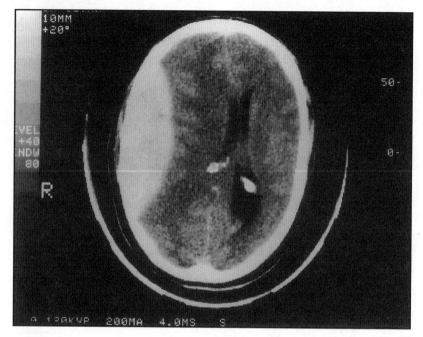

Fig. 2.4

(a) What is the diagnosis?

(b) What is the most probable cause?

(c) What are the main principles involved in managing this case?

(d) What is cerebral perfusion pressure?

(e) What causes secondary brain injury?

STATION 2.5

You have an 8-year-old boy booked for an appendicectomy. His mother is very worried that his older brother ended up in ITU with a very high temperature after an appendicectomy.

How would you manage the situation?

STATION 2.6

(a) Describe the principles of the capnograph.

(b) What information can be gleaned from this piece of equipment?

STATION 2.7

A 78-year-old man is having a TURP done under spinal block. After an hour's operating he becomes confused and has a seizure.

(a) What is the diagnosis?

(b) How would you confirm the suspected diagnosis?

(c) How will you manage the situation?

STATION 2.8

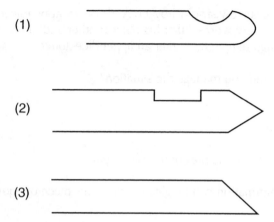

(1)

(2)

(3)

Fig. 2.8

(a) Name these needles

(b) Describe their major differences.

(c) What are the advantages of the various needles?

(d) What is the disadvantage of (b)?

(e) What factors influence post dural puncture headache?

(f) Explain the management for post dural puncture headache

STATION 2.9

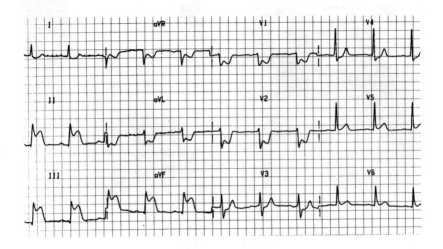

Fig. 2.9

Here is an ECG of a patient who complains of post-operative chest pain

(a) What does the ECG show?

(b) What is the diagnosis?

STATION 2.10

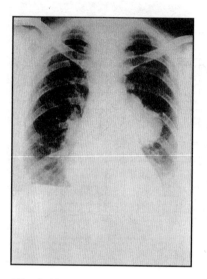

Fig. 2.10a

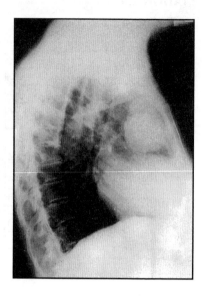

Fig. 2.10b

These are the PA and lateral CXRs of a 45-year-old lady who has presented for an elective operation.

(a) What does the chest X-ray show?

(b) What is the likely underlying diagnosis?

(c) What is myasthenia gravis?

(d) What medications and other treatments are there for this condition?

(e) What are the anaesthetic implications of myasthenia gravis?

STATION 2.11

A 68-year-old smoker is admitted for an elective operation. He is found on routine blood tests to have a haemoglobin of 19 g/dl.

(a) What is the likely diagnosis?

(b) Why is the haemoglobin elevated?

(c) What other condition is he likely to suffer from?

STATION 2.12

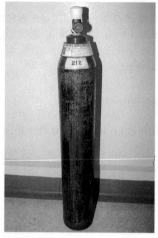

Fig. 2.12

(a) What are the concentrations of the various gases in this cylinder?

(b) What is the pressure within a full cylinder?

(c) Is this useful for an acute attack of bronchospasm?

(d) In what clinical scenario is it useful?

(e) How does it work in that situation?

(f) What physics principles explain this?

STATION 2.13

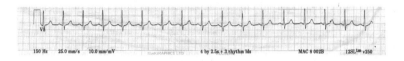

Fig. 2.13

You attend a cardiac arrest at which there is no cardiac output despite the above ECG trace.

(a) What is the diagnosis?

(b) What are the potentially reversible causes for this?

STATION 2.14

A 20-year-old West African male is admitted for urgent appendicectomy. A routine full blood count reveals a haemoglobin of 9.5 g/dl. He denies any relevant past medical history.

(a) What might be the cause of his low haemoglobin?

(b) How would you investigate it?

STATION 2.15

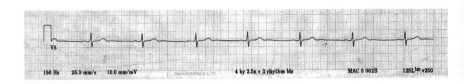

Fig. 2.15

(a) What does the ECG show?

(b) When and with what might you treat it?

(c) What are the likely causes of this ECG?

STATION 2.16

A 26-year-old male has had an arthroscopy as a day case. He insists on going home afterwards, but admits that he lied beforehand about there being someone at home.

How would you discuss the matter with him?

PRACTICE EXAMINATION 2: VIVA

Viva 2a

PHARMACOLOGY
Local anaesthetics

What is a local anaesthetic agent?

How does benzocaine work?

In what way does inflammation affect local anaesthetic efficacy? Why?

What is the problem with bupivacaine? What role does the racemic mixture play in this problem? What is the maximum recommended 'safe dose' of bupivacaine?

What isomers does one encounter with bupivacaine? Which is the safer?

PHYSIOLOGY
Nephron

How does the nephron work?

Viva 2b

CLINICAL

A previously fit and well 30-year-old male sustains an isolated femoral fracture following a road traffic accident.
On admission he appears well. His pulse rate is 100/min and blood pressure 110/70.
His Glasgow Coma Scale score is 15.
Six hours after admission he becomes acutely dyspnoeic.

What are the likely causes for his deterioration?

How would you manage him?

This man is found to have suffered a fat embolus.

What investigations would you perform, what would they be likely to show and how would you manage him?

PHYSICS
Rotameters

What is a rotameter?

What safety devices are employed in flowmeters?

2.1   **Answers: A B D E**

The dextrans are a group of branched polysaccharides produced by bacterial modification of sucrose. They improve peripheral blood flow by reducing blood viscosity and adhering to both the endothelium and cellular elements of blood, thus causing problems with the cross matching of blood. Impairing platelet activity as well as reducing levels of factor VIII reduces the risk of venous thrombosis. Side-effects include renal failure due to tubular obstruction in the kidney and anaphylactoid reactions, thought to be the result of previous cross-immunisation against bacterial antigens.

2.2   **Answers: A D**

Potassium is an intracellular ion released from myocytes during depolarisation following suxamethonium and raising the serum K transiently by 0.5 mmol/l in normal adults. Extensive tissue trauma will also release potassium from the cells, raising serum levels. Metabolic alkalosis will cause hypokalaemia following renal compensation. D-tubocurarine, being a non-depolarising neuromuscular blocking agent, has no effect on serum K.

2.3   **Answers: A E**

Non-depolarising neuromuscular blocking agents are highly ionised compounds at body pH, exhibiting two quaternary ammonium groups. Their action is prolonged by hypothermia and severe acidosis. Monitoring of the blockade exhibits fade during 'train of four', tetanic contraction also exhibits fade followed by post tetanic facilitation. Depolarising neuromuscular blockade produces fasciculations and may exhibit dual block.

2.4

Answers: A D E

Although not generally available in the UK, ether is still used world-wide. It is considered one of the safest of inhalational anaesthetics, largely as cardiovascular depression is late and is preceded by respiratory depression. However, postoperative convulsions often associated with pyrexia and prior atropine administration are recognised.

Once serum levels of bupivacaine exceed 2–4 mg/ml, either by misplacement of solution or excess dosage, central nervous system depression followed by convulsions may occur. Concurrently, there may be cardiovascular collapse. Suxamethonium produces muscle fasciculation and inhalational anaesthetics may all produce post-operative shivering, which is not to be confused with convulsions.

2.5

Answers: A B

Pain is not associated with intravenous injection of thiopentone, but should raise the possibility of intra-arterial injection or extravasation of the drug, both of which cause a severe burning sensation. Severe hypotension may occur especially following relative overdose or during hypovolaemia. Respiratory depression is common. Thiopentone induces liver enzymes but liver toxicity has not been reported.

2.6

Answers: A C D E

The boiling point of enflurane is 56.5°C compared with 50°C of halothane. Hypotension is more common with enflurane than halothane, due to greater myocardial depression and peripheral vasodilation. Halothane causes greater sensitisation of the myocardium and therefore arrhythmias. Respiratory depression is greater with enflurane reducing tidal volume and increasing respiratory rate. Both agents will release inorganic fluoride ions though the amount from halothane is negligible.

2.7

Answer: A

Digoxin is widely used to treat supraventricular arrhythmias such as atrial fibrillation (AF), atrial flutter and supraventricular tachycardia (SVT). Ventricular tachyarrhythmias are a feature of digoxin toxicity, which may be treated with phenytoin or digoxin specific antibodies.

2.8   **Answers: A C**

Propranolol is a non-selective competitive antagonist at β_1 and β_2 receptors. It will therefore result in bronchoconstriction and reduced cardiac output in patients with bronchial hypersensitivity or cardiac impairment. By blocking β_1 receptors it slows heart rate and may be used either alone or in conjunction with digoxin to slow the ventricular response in atrial fibrillation.

2.9   **Answers: A B C**

Dopamine is a naturally occurring catecholamine and neuro-transmitter found in postganglionic sympathetic nerve endings and in the adrenal medulla. Its effects are dose-dependent. In doses up to 5 μg/kg/min renal blood flow, GFR, urine output and sodium excretion (by impaired tubular reabsorption of Na^+ ions) are increased. At 10 μg/kg/min peripheral resistance is increased due to an action on alpha adrenoreceptors. Although tachycardia is common, ventricular arrhythmias usually only occur at very high doses.

2.10   **Answers: A D E**

A derivative of phencyclidine, ketamine is metabolised in the liver to weakly active metabolites which are excreted in the urine. Ketamine increases blood pressure and heart rate as well as cerebral blood flow and intra-cranial pressure (ICP). Muscular tone is enhanced as is uterine tone. Airway reflexes are maintained and, as salivation may be increased, pre-medication with an anti-sialagogue is recommended.

2.11   **Answers: C D E**

Sodium dantrolene is a skeletal muscle relaxant that directly effects excitation-contraction coupling within skeletal muscle by reducing the amount of calcium released by the sarcoplasmic reticulum. It has no effect on neuromuscular transmission, the membrane potential or muscle excitability itself. It is effective in treating malignant hyperpyrexia at a dose of 1–10 mg/kg.

2.12   **Answers: A E**

Isoflurane was first synthesised in 1965 along with its isomer enflurane, but not introduced until 1980 because of (subsequently unfounded) reports of carcinogenicity in rats. Its MAC is 1.15 and SVP at 20°C is 33 kPa; similar to halothane (32 kPa). Blood pressure is reduced mainly by peripheral vasodilation, but at 1 MAC or less cerebral blood flow is not increased.

2.13

Answers: A C

Blood pressure and systemic vascular resistance are reduced by morphine mediated by histamine release. Miosis results from stimulation of the Edinger–Westphal nucleus and vomiting from stimulation of the chemoreceptor trigger zone in the floor of the IVth ventricle. Although there is a reduced ventilatory response to hypoxia and hypercapnia, at normal therapeutic dosages the arterial pCO_2 is not markedly raised.

2.14

Answers: A B C D E

The pharmacological effects of chlorpromazine are mediated by antagonism of histamine receptors, alpha adrenergic receptors, central D2 dopaminergic receptors, muscarinic cholinergic receptors and serotoninergic receptors.

2.15

Answers: B D E

Chlorpropamide is a sulphonylurea, which stimulates insulin release from pancreatic B cells and increases the number and sensitivity of peripheral insulin receptors. It is extensively metabolised by the liver to a variety of active and inactive metabolites which are renally excreted. The elimination half-life of 27–39 hours may be markedly increased by renal impairment. Side-effects occur in around 6% of patients (compared with 3% of those taking tolbutamide) and include a disulfiram-like interaction when taken with alcohol.

2.16

Answers: A B E

The MAC of an inhalation anaesthetic agent, expressed in terms of % of one atmosphere, serves as a useful guide to clinical dosage as potency is inversely related to MAC. Potency is related to the oil/gas partition coefficient. MAC is reduced by other depressant drugs, including other anaesthetic agents, hypothermia, hypoxaemia and extremes of age. It is unaffected by sex, acid-base balance and hyper or hypocapnia.

2.17

Answers: A B C D E

Halothane produces a dose-dependent decrease in myocardial contractility and cardiac output mediated by inhibition of Ca ion flux within myocardial cells. The systemic vascular resistance is decreased by 15–18% and the baroreceptor reflexes are obtunded. It has ganglion blocking and central vasomotor depressant actions all resulting in hypotension.

2.18   **Answers: B E**

Bupivacaine is a local anaesthetic which acts by diffusing through neural sheaths in the uncharged base form to combine with hydrogen ions forming a cationic structure which is able to block the internal opening of the sodium ion channel thereby preventing Na ion conductance and cell membrane depolarisation. The recommended maximal dose is 2 mg/kg. Metabolism occurs in the liver by N-dealkylation. Methaemoglobinaemia occurs with > 600 mg administration of prilocaine.

2.19   **Answers: A B C E**

Chlorpropamide is an oral hypoglycaemic agent and has no anticonvulsant properties. Benzodiazepines and chlormethiazole act via facilitation of GABA receptors, opening chloride channels and hyperpolarising the cell membrane. Barbiturates also enhance chloride ion conductance but in the absence of GABA receptors.

2.20   **Answers: A D E**

Albumin is synthesised in the liver and forms a major constituent of plasma protein. It is important in maintenance of the plasma oncotic pressure. Normal values are 34–45 g/l. The plasma concentration is reduced in severe illness, infection, trauma, chronic liver disease and malabsorption.

2.21   **Answers: B E**

Neither atropine nor methylene blue cause methaemoglobinaemia. Prilocaine in doses in excess of 600 mg may cause methaemoglobinaemia. Levels of methaemoglobin should be monitored when using nitric oxide in ARDS patients. Cyanide ions will react with methaemoglobin to form cyanomethaemoglobin i.e. they will reduce levels of methaemoglobin.

2.22   **Answers: A C E**

Cyclizine is thought to exert its anti-emetic action via blockade of H_1 receptors centrally whilst hyoscine acts via antagonism of acetylcholine at muscarinic receptors. Perphenazine blocks D2 dopaminergic receptors whereas apomorphine, an alkaloid derived from morphine, has powerful dopamine agonist action causing intense stimulation of the chemoreceptor trigger zone and vomiting. Carbimazole inhibits thyroxine synthesis.

2.23   **Answers: A B C D E**

Although thiazide diuretics act mainly on the distal convoluted tubule, where they inhibit Na ion reabsorption, they also act at the proximal convoluted tubule causing weak inhibition of carbonic anhydrase and increasing bicarbonate and potassium excretion. Side-effects include hypokalaemia, hyponatraemia, hyper-uricaemia, hypomagnesaemia, hypochloraemia, hyperglycaemia, hyperchloraemic alkalosis and hypercholesterolaemia. Whilst loop diuretics promote calcium excretion and are used in the treatment of hypercalcaemia, thiazide diuretics cause calcium retention and increased serum calcium levels. Due to the effects on serum potassium and magnesium levels they may potentiate digoxin and increase the likelihood of digoxin toxicity.

2.24   **Answers: C D E**

Ketamine causes tachycardia, an increase in blood pressure, central venous pressure and cardiac output secondary to an increase in sympathetic tone. Cerebral blood flow, intraocular and intracerebral pressure are all increased. Emergence delirium and hallucinations are common and reduced by benzodiazepine premedication. Muscle hypertonia may require positioning of the patient prior to induction.

2.25   **Answers: A C E**

The effect of systemic or respiratory acidosis is to increase the potency and prolong the duration of action of non-depolarising neuromuscular blocking drugs. This may be either due to a direct effect of the pH on the physiochemical properties of these drugs or due to the concurrent effects on potassium metabolism; alkalosis promoting a shift of potassium into the cells raising the resting membrane potential and preventing depolarisation. Both hypermagnesaemia and hypocalcaemia will potentiate a competitive neuromuscular blockade due to their effects on the membrane potential.

2.26   **Answers: A C D**

Five cyanide ions are produced by the degradation of each nitroprusside molecule; one reacts with methaemoglobin to form cyanomethaemoglobin, the four remaining cyanide molecules enter the plasma, 80% of these react with thiosulphate in a reaction catalysed by hepatic rhodanese to form inactive thiocyanate. The remainder react with hydroxycobalamin to form cyanocobalamin. When these pathways are exhausted free cyanide ions are able to bind to cytochrome C, inhibiting aerobic metabolism and resulting in lactic acidosis. Toxicity is related to the rate of infusion rather than the total dose used, however it is recommended that no more than 1.5 mg/kg is infused acutely.

2.27   **Answers: B C**

Propranolol may mask the symptoms of hypoglycaemia but does not cause it *per se*. It is a competitive antagonist at β_1 and β_2 receptors resulting in bradycardia and bronchoconstriction. Adrenergic receptor activity is mediated via cyclic AMP as is enoximone, which is a phosphodiesterase inhibitor.

2.28   **Answers: B C D**

Frusemide acts by inhibition of active chloride ion reabsorption in the proximal tubule and ascending limb of the loop of Henle. By reducing the tonicity of the renal medulla, a hypotonic or isotonic urine is produced. This results in a diuresis and contraction of the circulating blood volume.

2.29   **Answers: B D**

Digoxin, verapamil and adenosine are used for supraventricular tachycardias, their site of action being the atrioventricular node. Disopyramide acts at the level of the atria, ventricles and accessory pathways whereas lignocaine acts on the ventricles only. Both can be used to treat ventricular tachycardia.

2.30
Answers: A B

It is the partial pressure of an anaesthetic agent in the brain which is responsible for its anaesthetic effect. If an agent is insoluble in blood, little is removed from the alveoli by the pulmonary circulation and therefore the alveolar and brain partial pressure will rise rapidly. For agents with a high solubility large amounts are removed from the alveoli, increasing ventilation ensures a rapid replacement of the agent and increases the speed of induction. An increased cardiac output results in greater pulmonary blood flow, increasing uptake of the agent and therefore lowering alveolar partial pressure. Conversely, a low cardiac output will result in a reduced peripheral blood flow and blood returning to the lungs will still contain some anaesthetic agent. The partial pressure gradient between alveoli and blood is reduced, the net result being that alveolar concentration rises more rapidly.

2.31
Answers: A B C

In primary adrenal failure (Addison's disease) the anterior pituitary secretes adrenocorticotrophic hormone in response to stimulation by corticotrophin releasing factor from the hypothalamus, but no cortisol or aldosterone is produced by the adrenal glands. ACTH, being similar to melatonin, produces hyperpigmentation of the skin creases. Lack of cortisol and aldosterone results in hypovolaemia, hyponatraemia, hypoglycaemia, hyperkalaemia and hypercalcaemia. Treatment is with cortisol and aldosterone replacement therapy.

2.32
Answers: A B D E

Angiotensin II is produced from the action of angiotensin converting enzyme on angiotensin I in the lungs. It is a potent arteriolar vasoconstrictor which directly stimulates the thirst centre and releases aldosterone from the adrenal gland. The half-life of angiotensin II is 1–2 minutes and it is metabolised throughout the body including the lungs by a series of enzymes called angiotensinase.

2.33
Answers: B E

Gastrin is produced by the G cells in the lateral walls of the glands in the antral portion of the gastric mucosa. It is released in response to intra-luminal peptides or distension and vagal stimulation, which is mediated by gastrin releasing peptide and not acetylcholine. Adrenaline due to sympathetic stimulation stimulates gastrin secretion and intraluminal acid provides the negative feedback loop to inhibit further gastrin production.

2.34
Answers: A C

Clearance is a calculated figure representing complete removal of a substance from plasma by passage through an organ, usually the kidney. In order to measure renal plasma flow the Fick principle may be applied. Since PAH is almost completely cleared by the kidney during one passage it is used to calculate renal plasma flow by determining steady state plasma and urine concentrations. Creatinine not urea is used to determine GFR, as following filtration it is not reabsorbed nor secreted by the tubular cells. Inulin is filtered by the nephron but neither secreted nor reabsorbed, unlike glucose which is completely reabsorbed unless the renal threshold is exceeded. Water is reabsorbed in the distal collecting ducts under the control of ADH.

2.35
Answers: A C D

Physiological dead space equals anatomical plus alveolar dead space. The anatomical dead space comprises nose, mouth, pharynx and large airways not lined by respiratory epithelium. It is affected by posture, the size of the patient and increases with large respiratory efforts due to traction exerted on the bronchus by surrounding lung parenchyma. Alveolar dead space comprises of the areas of the lung that are ventilated but not perfused.

2.36
Answer: D

Surfactant is produced by type II pneumocytes and forms a thin layer over the alveoli reducing the surface tension and increasing the compliance of the lung. One of the constituents of surfactant; dipalmitoyl phosphatidyl choline (DPPC) has hydrophobic and hydrophilic areas within the molecule which align themselves over the surface of the alveolus to exert their action.

2.37

Answers: B C D E

The pyramidal system consists of fibres running from area IV in the motor cortex to the contralateral motor nerves. The fibres form the pyramids in the medulla from where they gain their name and at which level 80–90% decussate to form the lateral corticospinal tract of the spinal cord.

2.38

Answer: E

Both cardiac and smooth muscle cells, but not skeletal muscle, have low resistance bridges between individual cells allowing them to act in a syncytial fashion. The resting membrane potential of skeletal and cardiac muscle is similar at –90 mV but smooth muscle has a much higher and more variable resting potential. The action potential duration is around 200 ms in cardiac muscle but shorter in smooth and skeletal muscle. Calcium influx from extra cellular fluid is important in smooth muscle contraction, whereas in skeletal and cardiac myocytes calcium is released from the sarcoplasmic reticulum.

2.39

Answers: B C D E

The pulmonary vascular system is a distensible, low pressure system. Pulmonary arterial pressure is around 25/9 mm Hg with a mean pressure of 15 mm Hg. In the normal erect subject 9% of the blood volume is in the pulmonary circulation, but this increases to 16% in the supine subject. Pulmonary vascular resistance is increased by adrenergic agonists, angiotensin II, thromboxanes and hypoxia. During exercise, pulmonary artery pressure is increased as is pulmonary blood flow; vascular resistance falls as previously closed portions of the vascular bed are recruited.

2.40

Answers: All false

Due to the patent ductus arteriosus and foramen ovale, the left and right heart sides of the heartpump in parallel in the fetus. At birth the systemic vascular resistance suddenly rises, the infant gasps producing negative intrathoracic pressures of –40 to 50 cm H_2O. Pulmonary vascular resistance falls and blood is pumped around the pulmonary circulation. Blood returning from the lungs raises the pressure in the left atrium, closing the foramen ovale and separating the two circulations. The ductus arteriosus constricts at birth and fuses completely within the first few days of life. Haemoglobin F persists until 3–4 months of age.

2.41   **Answers: B C D E**

Carbon dioxide is carried in the blood mainly as bicarbonate; 5–10% dissolved in plasma and 5–30% as carbamino compounds. It is 20 times more soluble than oxygen and therefore crosses the placenta more easily. Deoxygenated haemoglobin can bind more carbon dioxide to form carbamino compounds thus facilitating loading of CO_2 in the peripheral capillaries.

2.42   **Answers: C E**

Emotional syncope is commonly due to abrupt vasodilatation combined with a reflex bradycardia. Sinus arrhythmia causes an increased heart rate on inspiration and slowing on expiration. Noradrenaline infusion causes a bradycardia via increased blood pressure feeding back via the carotid sinus stretch receptors.

2.43   **Answer: A**

The carotid and to a lesser extent aortic bodies respond to reduced partial pressure (rather than content) of oxygen in arterial blood by stimulating ventilation. The central chemoreceptors respond to changes in pH and pCO_2, whilst the central respiratory neurones are depressed by hypoxia.

2.44   **Answer: A**

Muscle fibres are long multinucleate cells 50–70 μm in diameter and ranging in length from a few millimetres to a few centimetres. Individual fibres have a single neural contact near the mid-point, from where the action potential travels along the sarcolemmal membrane and down the transverse tubules to initiate a contraction.

2.45   **Answers: A C D**

The dorsal root is also called the sensory root because it carries only sensory fibres. Neurones from peripheral sensory receptors enter the spinal cord via the dorsal horn. Two-thirds of these neurones synapse in the dorsal grey horn of the spinal cord, the other third pass up the cord to the gracile and cuneate nuclei. Sensory neurones form part of the pathway for reflex arcs and the monitoring of muscular tone via the muscle spindles. The preganglionic output to the autonomic nervous system travels in the ventral nerve root.

2.46
Answers: C D E

Haemoglobin is a protein made up of 4 subunits, each of which contains a haem moiety which may bind reversibly with oxygen. Nearly all of the oxygen in blood is carried by red blood cells bound to haem. At 37°C the solubility of oxygen in plasma is 0.03 ml/l per mm Hg partial pressure. This equates to approximately 0.3 ml of O_2 per 100 ml of plasma. Plasma is 1.8 times as viscous as water but the major determinant of blood viscosity is the haematocrit. Plasma skimming occurs when red cells tend to flow in the centre of vessels leaving relatively red cell poor blood at the periphery. 95% of the glucose consumed by red blood cells is metabolised by anaerobic glycolysis.

2.47
Answers: A B C E

The carotid bodies are found bilaterally at the bifurcation of the internal and external carotid arteries. They are supplied with blood by a branch of the external carotid artery. The rich blood supply of 200 ml/100 g/min (compared with 84 ml/100 g/min for the myocardium) is so great that the AVO$_2$ difference is very small and capillary gas tensions are very close to those of the arterial system. They respond to hypoxia, a rise in pCO_2 or H^+ concentration by stimulating respiration.

2.48
Answers: C D

At the onset of the Valsalva manoeuvre the rise in intrathoracic pressure compresses the central veins, reducing preload and cardiac output. Baroreceptor output is inhibited resulting in a tachycardia and increased peripheral vascular resistance.

2.49
Answers: C D E

CSF contains 50–60% of blood glucose, has lower pH than blood but will reflect changes in blood H^+ concentration. 70% of CSF is formed by the choroid plexuses and absorbed via bulk flow into the arachnoid villi and cerebral blood vessels. Increased venous pressure will reduce the reabsorptive capacity.

2.50   **Answers: B C**

The ABO blood groups are inherited in a Mendelian fashion. Donated blood is separated from plasma and resuspended in another medium prior to transfusion.

The characteristics of each blood group are as follows.

Phenotype	Genotype	Antigen on cells	Antibody in serum	Frequency
A	AA, AO	A	Anti B	42%
B	BB, BO	B	Anti A	8%
AB	AB	A, B	None	3%
O	OO	None	Anti A, Anti B	47%

2.51   **Answer: A**

Acetylcholine is the transmitter at nicotinic receptors of the neuromuscular junction. Formed within the nerve terminal from choline and acetyl coenzyme A in the presence of choline transferase, it is released into the synaptic cleft where it is later hydrolysed by acetylcholinesterase. Botulinum toxin binds irreversibly to the nerve ending preventing acetylcholine release.

2.52   **Answer: A**

Enkephalin is an endogenous pentapeptide opioid agonist formed from proencephalon. It is found in the nerve endings of the gastrointestinal tract, adrenal, medulla and many different parts of the brain. It has a short half-life in the brain, terminated by metabolism by enkephalinase enzymes. Pro-opiomelanocortin the precursor of endorphin is primarily located in the hypothalamus and pituitary.

2.53   **Answers: B C D**

Tachycardia and an increase in the force of myocardial contraction are both due to β_1 adrenergic agonism, mediated by increases in intracellular cAMP. Pupillary dilation is mediated via alpha agonism which also produces vasoconstriction of splanchnic and visceral vessels. Vasodilatation in muscle and skin vessel beds is mediated via β_2 and some β_1 receptors.

2.54   **Answers: B E**

Glucocorticoids cause protein catabolism and increased hepatic glycogenesis and gluconeogenesis. They have mild mineralo-corticoid activity promoting K^+ loss and retaining salt and water. They affect bone by promoting resorption and inhibiting formation resulting in osteoporosis. Although cortisol feeds back on the anterior pituitary inhibiting ACTH secretion, it does not depress other functions of the pituitary gland.

2.55   **Answers: B D**

Isotonic saline has the same osmolality as plasma and will cause plasma expansion without changing osmolality. Vasopressin reduces osmolality via water retention whilst aldosterone will increase osmolality via Na^+ retention from sweat and salivary glands and in the kidney. Isotonic glucose will be rapidly metabolised resulting in a reduction in osmolality. 20% albumin solution is hypertonic, drawing 3 times the administered volume into the circulation within 15 minutes.

2.56   **Answers: A B C D E**

Within a few minutes of TSH injection iodide binding is increased in the thyroid gland. Formation of T3, T4 and iodotyrosines are increased as well as secretion of thyroglobulin into the colloid. TSH affects its action via G proteins and cAMP.

2.57   **Answer: E**

Due to failure of exocrine and endocrine functions of the pancreas, both insulin and glucagon will decrease, impairing carbohydrate and fat metabolism and increasing plasma levels of free fatty acids. Steatorrhoea is common due to the lack of pancreatic lipase.

2.58   **Answers: A C**

Glucagon is glycogenolytic, gluconeogenetic, lipolytic and ketogenic. Glucose is formed from amino acids thus lowering plasma levels whilst free fatty acids are released. It exerts a positive inotropic and chronotropic action on the myocardium via increased myocardial calcium release and has been used in the treatment of β adrenergic antagonist overdoses, though it does not stimulate the sympathetic nervous system directly.

2.59   **Answers: A B**

Both vasopressin and renin are secreted in response to a reduced extracellular fluid volume. Progesterone blocks the action of aldosterone. ACTH and thyroxine are unaffected.

2.60   **Answer: E**

High plasma calcium reduces intestinal absorption via reduction in 1,25 dihydroxycholecalciferol and formation of 24,25 dihydroxy-cholecalciferol instead. Calcitonin is increased inhibiting bone reabsorption and increasing urinary Ca^{++} excretion. Bone demineralisation may occur in the presence of primary hyper-parathyroidism but is not directly due to hypercalcaemia itself.

2.61   **Answers: A D**

The Wright's respirometer is a vane anemometer. It measures volume by monitoring the continuous rotation of the vane as it is moved by the passing gas. It tends to over-read at high tidal volumes and under-read at low volumes as a result of the inertia of the vanes. Moisture will cause the vanes to stick resulting in inaccurate readings.

2.62   **Answers: A C D**

The use of evoked potentials for monitoring the depth of anaesthesia or the integrity of the central nervous system during surgery involves monitoring the electrical activity produced by repetitive peripheral or central stimulation. Somatosensory, auditory and visual evoked potentials have all been used but they require complex equipment to increase the recording sensitivity and reduce background interference. Somatosensory evoked potentials involve supra-maximal stimulation usually of the tibialis or median nerves with simultaneous recording over the sensory area appropriate to the site of stimulation. Transmission is altered in the form of latency and amplitude of the signal with varying levels of anaesthesia.

2.63   **Answers: A D**

For accurate measurement of blood pressure it is essential that the width of the cuff should be in proportion to the size of the arm. The correct width is 20% greater than the width of the arm. Raising the arm above the level of the heart will result in a lower pressure being recorded. Slow cuff deflation and the position of the sphygmomanometer will not affect the reading.

2.64
Answer: B
Nitrogen at high pressure has a narcotic effect and this is the reason for the use of helium for diving to depths below 70 m. During normal respiration, with laminar gas flow, it is the viscosity of a gas that determines flow, however the viscosity of helium and nitrogen are similar. During turbulent flow the density of a gas becomes important; helium is less dense than nitrogen and it is for this reason that it is used as a carrier gas in cases of upper airway obstruction.

2.65
Answers: A B E
A current of as little as 150 micro amps delivered direct to the myocardium can induce ventricular fibrillation. The risk of electric current flowing along an intracardiac catheter is increased if it is filled with a conducting solution such as saline, likewise an oesophageal electrode can provide a low resistance route for the delivery of current to the myocardium. Multiple earth loops will increase the likelihood of current flowing through the patient from any faulty equipment. Connection of equipment casing to earth, double insulation of conducting wire within equipment and the use of isolated circuits are all measures taken to try to avoid microshock.

2.66
Answers: A C
The Fick principle relates blood flow to an organ in unit time to the amount of marker substance taken up by that organ in that time and the concentration difference of the substance in vessels supplying and draining the organ. For cardiac output the oxygen consumption by the lungs together with arterial and mixed venous oxygen contents are used.

$$\text{Cardiac output (l/min)} = \frac{O_2 \text{ consumption (ml/min)}}{\text{arterial-mixed venous } O_2 \text{ concentration (ml/l)}}$$

2.67   **Answers: A B E**

Nitrous oxide is produced by heating ammonium nitrate above 240°C. Ammonia, nitric acid, nitrogen, nitric oxide and nitrogen dioxide are also produced. Ammonia and nitric acid reconstitute to form ammonium nitrate; nitric oxide and nitrogen dioxide pass through a series of scrubbers to ensure they are completely removed, as both are highly toxic. Carbon dioxide is formed by heating calcium or magnesium carbonate. Helium is obtained from natural gas. Oxygen concentrators compress and cool air then remove water vapour by passing through silicone gel and nitrogen by passing through zeolite filled cylinders. They can provide 90–95% oxygen at up to 4 l/min, however 2–5% argon is present in the final mixture.

2.68   **Answers: C D**

In an exponential process the rate of change of a quantity at any time is proportional to the quantity at that time. The half-life is the time taken for the initial quantity to fall to half its original value. The time constant is the time in which the process would have been completed had the initial rate of change continued unchanged. Consequently the time constant is longer than the half-life. After one time constant 63% of the change is completed leaving 37% remaining.

2.69   **Answers: A B C E**

Airway resistance is the pressure difference between the alveoli and the mouth divided by the flow rate. Mouth pressure can be measured using a water filled manometer and alveolar pressure can be deduced from measurements made in a body plethysmograph. Airway resistance is increased at low lung volumes due to the reduction of radial traction produced by the lung parenchyma. Thus airway resistance is increased by anaesthesia due to reduced lung volume though inhalational anaesthetics *per se* reduce resistance via a bronchodilator action. Positive end expiratory pressure will increase lung volume and reduce airway resistance.

2.70   **Answers: A E**

The single breath nitrogen test is used to measure anatomical dead space by following nitrogen concentration at the mouth after a single inspiration of 100% oxygen. N_2 concentration rises as dead space gas is increasingly washed out by alveolar gas. Pure alveolar gas forms a plateau concentration of nitrogen, then towards the end of expiration an abrupt increase in N_2 concentration is seen. This is the closing volume caused by preferential emptying of the apex of the lung, which has a relatively higher N_2 concentration. Distribution of gas delivery in the lung is measured with xenon and diffusion capacity with carbon monoxide.

2.71   **Answers: A C D E**

The alveolar arterial gradient is an indicator of the exchange properties of the lung. It depends on diffusion across the alveolar membrane and physiological shunt. If the closing capacity exceeds the functional residual capacity there will be increased V/Q mismatch and shunting. In the elderly the closing capacity rises often exceeding the functional residual capacity during normal tidal volume breathing, resulting in V/Q mismatch.

2.72   **Answers: B C D**

Commercial oxygen is produced by fractional distillation of air. Its boiling point is –183°C and the critical temperature is –118°C. Exposure to hyperbaric oxygen produces increased oxygen dissolved in blood but no increase in the amount of oxygen carried by haemoglobin, which is usually almost fully saturated. Symptoms evoked by hyperbaric oxygen are tracheobronchial irritation, dizziness, nausea, ringing in the ears, convulsions and coma. Bone marrow depression occurs following prolonged exposure to nitrous oxide.

2.73   Answers: B C E

Nitrous oxide is a vapour at room temperature as this is below its critical temperature of 36.5°C. Nitrous oxide cylinders are filled with a combination of liquid and gaseous nitrous oxide. If completely filled with liquid any increase in temperature would cause a dangerous rise in pressure within the cylinder; therefore nitrous oxide cylinders are only partially filled with liquid according to the filling ratio. The pressure gauge relates to the amount of nitrous oxide in the gaseous phase, and is not therefore a reliable indicator of the amount remaining in the cylinder until all the liquid has been exhausted. Higher oxides of nitrogen are produced during the heating of ammonium nitrate to form nitrous oxide. They can be tested for with moistened starch-iodide paper, which will turn blue in the presence of nitric oxide or nitrogen dioxide.

2.74   Answers: C D E

The approximate composition of soda lime is 90% calcium hydroxide, 5% sodium hydroxide and 1% potassium hydroxide with silicates for binding and an indicator. The moisture content is 14–19%, which is essential for effective carbon dioxide absorption. Carbon dioxide in solution reacts with sodium and potassium hydroxide to form the respective carbonates, which then react with calcium hydroxide to produce calcium carbonate, replenishing sodium and potassium hydroxide. In a properly packed canister half the volume should be space between the granules. Heat is produced by the chemical reaction that takes place.

2.75   Answers: A B C

The Magill circuit is an example of a Mapleson type A, the coaxial modification of which is called the Lack circuit. The effort required to open the expiratory valve precludes its use in small children but it is suitable for those weighing more than 20 kg. During spontaneous ventilation exhaled dead space is retained, to be inhaled at the next inspiration, whereas exhaled alveolar gas is vented through the expiratory valve. Therefore fresh gas flow may be reduced to alveolar ventilation (normally about 70% of minute ventilation) before rebreathing will occur.

2.76   **Answers: A B C D**

The central venous pressure is usually measured with the patient lying flat, and expressed in cm H_2O above a fixed point level with the right atrium e.g. the mid axillary line. Alterations in the position of the patient will affect the measurement as will wetting the manometer tube plug. During normal spontaneous breathing the pressure falls on inspiration and rises on expiration. Large negative intrathoracic pressures such as those generated by patients with airway obstruction will accentuate the fall and cause inaccuracies in central venous pressure measurement.

2.77   **Answers: A B C D E**

Dirt on the bobbin or static electricity may cause the bobbin to stick to the glass tubing of the rotameter. Ventilators which exert back pressure such as the Manley will depress the level of the bobbin and errors of up to 7% may result. Rotameters are calibrated for an individual bobbin and a specific gas at sea level, changes in the type of gas or barometric pressure will lead to inaccuracy.

2.78   **Answers: A B D**

The critical temperature is defined as the temperature above which a substance cannot be liquefied however much pressure is applied. The critical pressure is the vapour pressure of a substance at its critical temperature. The word 'gas' applies to a substance above its critical temperature while 'vapour ' is the word used for a substance below its critical temperature. At room temperature oxygen and nitrogen are gases whilst nitrous oxide, carbon dioxide and halothane are vapours.

2.79   **Answer: D**

As the saturated vapour pressure is 152 mmHg then at atmospheric pressure (760 mmHg) the gas passing through the chamber will be approximately 20% saturated (152/760). As 2% of total gas flow passes through the chamber (80 ml/4L) then the inspired concentration is 0.4%.

2.80   **Answers: All false**

The critical pressure is the vapour pressure of a substance at its critical temperature.

2.81   **Answer: E**

The pressure within oxygen and entonox cylinders is 137 bar, nitrous oxide is stored at 40 bar. Entonox should not be stored at –8°C as this is below the pseudocritical temperature at which separation of the gases will occur allowing the possibility of delivering a hypoxic mixture of oxygen/nitrous oxide.

2.82   **Answers: B D**

According to the Hageni–Poiseuille equation regarding laminar flow:

$$\text{Gas flow} = \frac{\pi(P1 - P2)\ r^4}{8\mu l}$$

where P1 – P2 is the pressure drop, μ the viscosity and l the length of the tube. Density becomes important only in turbulent flow.

2.83   **Answers: A E**

The vapour pressure is the pressure exerted by molecules escaping from the surface of a liquid to enter the gaseous phase. When equilibrium is reached at any temperature, the number of molecules leaving the liquid equals the number re-entering it; the vapour pressure now equals the saturated vapour pressure (SVP). Raising the temperature increases the kinetic energy of the molecules allowing more to escape to the gaseous phase and raising the SVP. When SVP equals barometric pressure the liquid boils.

2.84   **Answers: A B C D E**

Fires and explosions occur when a substance combines with oxygen or other oxidising agent with the release of energy. Activation energy is required to start the process, which may be provided from sparks from electrical equipment or static electricity from clothing, shoes or work surfaces. The risk of accumulation of static electricity on walls and equipment is reduced if the relative humidity is kept high. Floors of operating theatres are made of conductive materials to allow any build up of static charge to be safely drained away.

2.85   **Answers: B E**

For an ideal gas, $PV = nRT$ where P is the pressure, V is volume, n is the number of moles of gas, R is the universal gas constant and T is temperature. Nitrous oxide is a vapour at room temperature. The contents of a cylinder of nitrous oxide at 40 bar are therefore a mixture of liquid and gas.

2.86   **Answers: B D E**

General anaesthesia inhibits the patients' ability to maintain body temperature by depressing the thermoregulatory centre in the hypothalamus. Conductive losses are of little importance in air, but become highly significant when water is the conducting medium. Respiratory losses account for 10% of heat loss of which 8% is due to the latent heat of vaporisation of water and 2% due to the heating of air. The temperature of a patient will rapidly fall following induction of general anaesthesia if no active warming measures are taken.

2.87   **Answers: B E**

Capnography is the continuous measurement and display of carbon dioxide in exhaled gas. It approximates to the alveolar partial pressure of carbon dioxide in normal subjects, however the normal $PaCO_2/PeCO_2$ gradient is 0.7 kPa and this will be increased by significant V/Q mismatch. Carbon dioxide absorbs infrared radiation within the sampling chamber of the capnograph. In the presence of nitrous oxide, carbon dioxide molecules may transfer some of this absorbed energy causing broadening of the absorption spectrum of nitrous oxide. Side stream capnographs withdraw a sample of exhaled gas from a connector at the patient's airway, resulting in a timing delay. Mainstream analysers are connected at the patient's airway and therefore have no transit time delay.

2.88   **Answers: B C E**

Diathermy is used to coagulate blood vessels and cut and destroy tissues during surgical procedures. It is the heating effect of a high density of current which causes this effect at the site of action. Normally high frequency (0.5–1.0 MHz) alternating current is used as lower frequencies are more likely to induce ventricular fibrillation. A sine wave pattern is used for cutting and a pulsed sine wave for coagulation. The current density is kept high at the site of intended damage, the forceps tips, but low at the large surface area plate which acts as the other electrode. Incorrect attachment of the plate may cause increased current density and burns in the area, or the current may escape via an alternative route such as via ECG electrodes.

2.89   **Answer: C**

$$Q = \frac{(P1 - P2)\ r^4\pi}{8\mu l}$$

According to the Hageni-Poiseuille equation, during conditions of laminar flow halving the diameter of the tube reduces the flow by one sixteenth (i.e. the fourth power) of its original value. Viscosity is inversely proportional to flow under these conditions. When the Reynold's number exceeds 2000 turbulent flow is likely. Under these conditions flow is no longer proportional to the pressure drop and the density of a fluid becomes an important factor in determining flow.

2.90   **Answers: A B C D E**

Damping of biological systems involves the progressive diminution of amplitude of oscillations in a resonant system. Excess damping, due to air bubbles, clots or kinking within the system results in a flattened trace. Optimal damping is defined as 0.6–0.7 of critical damping, producing a fast response without excessive oscillations. Using a shorter, stiffer, wider catheter may increase the resonant frequency of the system. Continuous flushing at rates of 3–4 ml/hr is preferable to intermittent flushing which may promote intimal damage and subsequent arterial thrombosis.

STATION 2.1

Answers and explanations

The cause of the abnormal chest radiograph is collapse/consolidation of the right middle lobe. This is most probably secondary to mucous plug obstruction. The diagnosis is confirmed on the lateral film (Fig. 2.1A).

In the middle lobe collapse, the horizontal fissure and lower half of the oblique fissure move towards one another – best seen in the lateral projection. Obscuration of the right heart border is often present, particularly when there is associated consolidation. Since the volume of the middle lobe is relatively small, indirect signs of volume loss, including elevation of the hemidiaphragm, mediastinal or hilar displacement and compensatory hyperinflation, are rarely present.

Each lobe collapses in a characteristic fashion (Figs. 2.1B and 2.1C) and radiological clues as to the cause of the collapse may be present, e.g. enlarged lymph nodes, bronchogenic carcinoma or an inhaled foreign body.

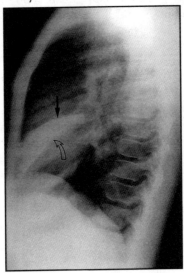

Fig. 2.1A

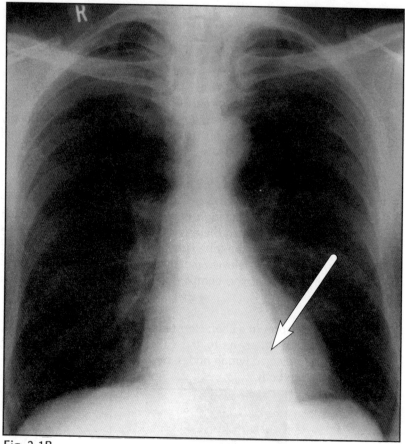

Fig. 2.1B

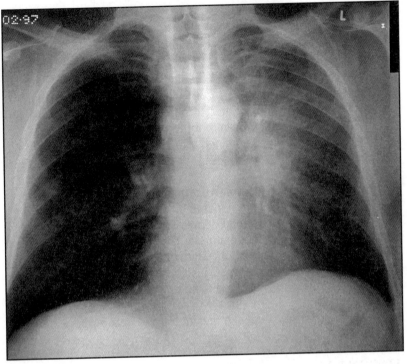

Fig. 2.1C

STATION 2.2

Answers and explanations

(a) The ECG shows a sinus bradycardia and the presence of J (junctional) waves, this suggests that the patient is suffering from hypothermia, possibly related to ingestion of alcohol, immersion in snow or cold water or immobility following, for example, a stroke. Hypothermia is defined as a core body temperature of < 35°C.

(b) J waves can be seen as small upstrokes at the junction of the S wave and ST segment; hence the name. Hypothermia is also associated with myocardial depression, hyperglycaemia and pancreatitis. As the temperature falls sinus bradycardia tends to give way to atrial fibrillation. Below 28°C VF may occur and finally asystole supervenes. Consciousness is depressed below 30°C and the pupils become fixed and dilated.

(c) Hypothermia is treated with rewarming and treating the arrhythmias.

STATION 2.3

Answers and explanations

(a) The arterial blood gas sample shows type 11 respiratory failure with hypoxia and carbon dioxide retention.

(b) Despite an elevated plasma bicarbonate the pH is acidotic, suggesting acute onchronic respiratory failure.

(c) The high bicarbonate is due to renal compensation for the chronic hypercarbia.

(d) The medical management involves oxygen therapy, steroids, nebulizers, antibiotics, physiotherapy and possibly aminophylline.

STATION 2.4

Answers and explanations

(a) The CT scan shows an extradural haematoma; the typically biconvex hypodense (white) area on the right.

(b) An extradural haematoma is classically due to a traumatic tear to the middle meningeal artery. Following initial loss of consciousness there may be a lucid interval followed by rapid decline into coma and a high mortality without surgical evacuation of the haematoma.

(c) The principles of neuroanaesthesia are that the blood pressure and the partial pressures of arterial oxygen and carbon dioxide should be kept within normal limits as these affect ICP and thus CPP too.

(d) Cerebral perfusion pressure (CPP) = Mean arterial pressure (MAP) – Intracranial pressure (ICP)

(e) Secondary brain injury is usually due to hypoxia.

STATION 2.5

Answer and explanation

The question implies that the brother had malignant hyperpyrexia (MH).

As MH is inherited as an autosomal dominant gene there is a reasonable chance that the patient is also MH susceptible.

There is clearly no time to refer him for muscle biopsy and caffeine and halothane contracture tests. Thus, he should be assumed to be MH susceptible and given an MH free anaesthetic.

The main trigger agents for MH are the volatile agents and suxamethonium.

As the SHO on call you must ask for senior assistance.

The mother should be reassured that her child can safely be given an anaesthetic without suffering the same problem as his older brother.

STATION 2.6

Answers and explanation

(a) The capnograph is used to monitor end-tidal carbon dioxide ($ETCO_2$). It employs the Luft principle which states that any molecule with two or more different atoms will absorb infra-red radiation. It is thus an infra-red spectrophotometer.

(b) The following information can be obtained from a capnograph.
   - Respiratory rate
   - Adequacy of ventilation
   - The $ETCO_2$ approximates to $PaCO_2$ which provides an assessment of adequacy of ventilation. Hypoventilation causes a raised $ETCO_2$; hyperventilation a reduced $ETCO_2$
   - Indirect assessment of cardiac output
     Presence of expired CO_2 ($ETCO_2$) depends on adequate lung perfusion which in turn depends on the cardiac output. In low cardiac output states the $ETCO_2$ will be low. In cardiac arrest there is no capnograph trace.
   - Disconnection alarm
     In the event of disconnection of breathing system/ventilator the capnograph trace will disappear
   - Confirmation of correct placement of ET tube
     The only reliable way of confirming tracheal placement of an ET tube is by a consistent, normal capnograph waveform
   - Detection of malignant hyperpyrexia
     In malignant hyperpyrexia the earliest signs are tachycardia, desaturation and an elevated and rising $ETCO_2$ (as well as temperature)
   - Detection of pulmonary embolus
     Pulmonary embolus (air, fat, cement, thrombosis) produces a sudden decline in $ETCO_2$ (in conjunction with desaturation and hypotension)
   - Indirect assessment of neuromuscular block
     In the absence of a peripheral nerve stimulator, the capnograph trace may indicate when the neuromuscular block wears off and the patient tries to breathe
   - Detection of breathing
     In, for example, inadequate fresh gas flow or exhausted soda lime in a circle system
   - Detection of bronchospasm
     The capnograph is altered in patients with chronic airflow limitation and also if bronchospasm develops intra-operatively

STATION 2.7

Answers and explanations

(a) The likely diagnosis is that this man has developed the TURP syndrome.
This is due to excessive absorption of irrigating fluid into the systemic circulation which leads to fluid overload, pulmonary oedema, hyponatraemia, confusion and convulsions.

(b) The diagnosis is confirmed by measuring the serum sodium.

(c) The management entails giving oxygen, frusemide and an anticonvulsant.

STATION 2.8

Answers and explanations

(a) These are (1) Sprotte, (2) Whitacre and (3) Quincke spinal needles.

(b) The major differences between these three types lies in the shape and bevel of their needle tips. The Quincke needle has a sharp (cutting), medium-bevel and a sharp (cutting) tip with end-injection. The Whitacre and Sprotte needles are known as atraumatic or non-cutting needles. The Sprotte needle has a bullet-shaped tip and the Whitacre needle has a pencil-point tip. They both have side-holes proximal to the tip, with the Sprotte needle having a more elongated lateral opening than that of the Whitacre needle.

(c) The advantage of the atraumatic (non-cutting) needles as their name suggests is that they cause less injury to the dura, separating the dural fibres leading to better dural closure after needle removal. This causes a smaller incidence of post-dural puncture headache (PDPH) compared with the Quincke needle.

(d) The Quincke needle tends to cut through the dural fibres causing a greater incidence of spinal leakage. This can be reduced by inserting the bevel of the Quincke needle parallel to the longitudinal dural fibres.

(e) Factors influencing PDPH
  - Gauge of spinal needle – the incidence of PDPH is proportional to the gauge
  - G or non-cutting spinal needle
  - Keeping bevel of cutting needle parallel to the dural fibres decreases the incidence
  - More common in young patients and in obstetric patients
  - Sex of patient – male patients have reduced incidence of PDPH

(f) Management of PDPH
Initially involves bedrest, hydration (aim for around 3 litres daily orally), regular simple analgesics and avoiding straining (consider laxatives). Methods to increase the epidural pressure such as the prone position and tight abdominal binders can be considered. Caffeine has been shown to relieve symptoms. Epidural blood patch should be performed after 1–3 days if the headache fails to respond to conservative treatment and is incapacitating. It should be performed early if the headache is severe. This involves taking 20 ml of fresh blood aseptically from the patient and injecting it into the epidural space. The epidural needle is ideally inserted at the same interspace at which the dural puncture occurred (if this is not possible the space below this is used). The whole 20 ml should be given epidurally unless discomfort is experienced before this. The patient lies supine for 30 minutes after this and is then allowed to mobilise. This procedure is over 90% successful with the first injection but occasionally a second blood patch is required.

STATION 2.9

Answers and explanation

(a) The ECG shows hyperacute ST segment elevation in the inferior leads; II, III and aVF.
There are reciprocal changes in aVR, aVL and leads V1–V2.

(b) These ECG changes indicate an acute inferior myocardial infarction. The diagnosis can be confirmed by documenting the typical pattern of cardiac enzyme rise over the following three days or by measuring the troponin-1 level.
The management is to give the patient oxygen, opiate analgesia and if not contraindicated by the recent surgery the patient should be thrombolysed.

STATION 2.10

Answers and explanations

(a) The PA chest X-ray shows a well circumscribed partly calcified mass at the upper left heart border. The lateral chest X-ray shows it to be an anterior mediastinal mass.

(b) The mass is a thymoma and the patient has myasthenia gravis.

(c) Myasthenia gravis is an autoimmune disease in which there are antibodies to the post-synaptic acetylcholine receptor of the neuromuscular junction. It results in weakness mainly of proximal limb, facial and eye muscles. It is associated with other autoimmune conditions and patients may have a thymoma.

(d) Management includes pharmacological treatment. Anticholinesterase drugs, such as pyridostigmine, increase the level of acetylcholine at the neuromuscular junction. An alternative approach is to use immunosuppressive agents such as azathioprine or steroids. Non-pharmacological treatments include plasmapheresis and thymectomy.

(e) The main consideration is the response of the patient to muscle relaxant. Patients are resistant to suxamethonium and exhibit unusual and sometimes prolonged blocks.

STATION 2.11

Answers and explanations

(a) The likely diagnosis is polycythaemia.
(b) This is likely to be a physiological response to chronic hypoxia. Alternatively he may have either polcythaemia rubra vera (PRV) or be secreting erythropoietin (EPO) from a tumour.
In PRV the platelets and white cells are also elevated and the patients often have splenomegaly and pruritus.
Hepatomas, massive uterine fibroids and adrenal tumours may secrete EPO.
In secondary polycythaemia the chronic hypoxia leads to increased renal production of EPO.
Venesection may be used to control the red cell mass.
In PRV drugs such as busulphan or cyclophosphamide are used to control the disease.
(c) He is a smoker and may well suffer from co-existent chronic obstructive airways disease.

STATION 2.12

Answers and explanations

(a) This is a heliox cylinder which contains 79% helium and 21% oxygen at 13 700 kPa or 137 bar.

(c) Helium/oxygen mixtures have a greater viscosity than nitrogen/oxygen mixtures. This is why helium is of little use in lower airway obstruction (e.g. asthma) where flow is laminar and therefore depends on viscosity rather than density.

(d) Heliox is useful in upper airway obstruction where turbulent flow occurs.

(e) This is because helium has a low density and density is an important determinant of turbulent flow. Thus a greater flow of heliox occurs than of a nitrogen/oxygen mixture as there is less airflow resistance and the work of breathing is decreased. It also makes turbulent flow less likely.

STATION 2.13

Answers and explanation

(a) The presence of a normal ECG trace in the absence of a cardiac output is electromechanical dissociation (EMD).

(b) The potentially reversible causes are:
The 4 Hs
- hypoxia
- hypo/hyperkalaemia
- hypovolaemia
- hypothermia

The 4 Ts
- tension pneumothorax
- cardiac tamponade
- thromboembolism
- toxic disturbance

STATION 2.14

Answers and explantions

(a) One diagnosis which should be excluded in someone of his ethnic origin, especially if he is febrile, is malaria. A thick and thin blood film to look for malarial parasites should be done.
A second possible diagnosis is sickle cell disease.
It is entirely possible that his low Hb may be due to iron deficiency or folate or vitamin B12 deficiency, though these would have less impact on his anaesthetic management.

(b) A reticulocyte count should be asked for along with a Sickledex test. If the Sickledex is positive then the amount of Hb S must be quantified by Hb electrophoresis. A simple blood film can be looked at for sickle red cells.
In the absence of any previous history it would be unusual, though not impossible, to get to the age of 20 and have homozygous sickle cell disease.
If he does have sickle cell disease he should be kept warm and well hydrated.
Tourniquets should be avoided as they may cause sickling in a limb.
Hypoxia and acidosis should be avoided.

STATION 2.15

Answers and explanation

(a) The ECG shows sinus bradycardia

(b) If the bradycardia causes cardiovascular compromise or is likely to lead to asystole then it should be treated with either intravenous atropine or glycopyrrolate.

(c) The causes include a patient who is very fit and athletic, β–blockers, hypothyroidism, vagal stimulation such as traction on the peritoneum or squint surgery.

STATION 2.16

Answers and explanations

Introduce yourself to the patient. Explain to him why it is important for him to have a responsible adult to escort him home and to be present for 24 hours post-operatively i.e. for safety reasons (his judgement may be impaired post-operatively) they may notice post-operative complications and are able to telephone for help should an adverse event occur. Ask him whether he can arrange for someone to escort him home and stay with him or stay at their home for 24 hours. If this is not possible then the patient will have to be admitted to a ward overnight. If the patient refuses to be admitted despite explanation of the reasons for this then this must be documented in the notes and a self-discharge form signed by the patient.

Viva 2a

PHARMACOLOGY
Local anaesthetics

What is a local anaesthetic agent?
A local anaesthetic is a substance that produces reversible blockade of peripheral nerve conduction.

How does benzocaine work?
Benzocaine works differently from other local anaesthetic agents. It is a non-ionised ester and is thought to block nerve conduction by causing membrane expansion and therefore distorting the sodium channels.

In what way does inflammation affect LA efficacy? Why?
Inflammation produces an acid environment making local anaesthetics less effective. At lower pH, local anaesthetics exist more in the ionised form. Only the unionised form of the local anaesthetics can diffuse through the cell membrane into the neurone, where they re-ionise and enter sodium ion channels to produce conduction blockade.
In addition, inflamed areas are more vascular and therefore any local anaesthetic used is more rapidly removed from the area.

What is the problem with bupivacaine? What role does the racemic mixture play in this problem? What is the maximum recommended 'safe dose' of bupivacaine?
Bupivacaine is much more cardiotoxic than other local anaesthetics. Ventricular arrhythmias and cardiac arrest are thought to be due to its effect on calcium and/or potassium channels (as well as sodium channels). Cardiac arrest due to bupivacaine toxicity may be very resistant to resuscitation. Massive doses of adrenaline have been shown to be effective in animal studies in this situation. Bretylium is thought to be of some use also.
The maximum recommended 'safe dose' of bupivacaine is 2 mg/kg.

What isomers does one encounter with bupivacaine? Which is the safer?
Bupivacaine has 2 isomers: R(+)-bupivacaine and S(-)-bupivacaine.

The R(+) enantiomer is 3–4 times more likely to cause cardiotoxicity than S(-)-bupivacaine in rabbit hearts. Less cardiovascular disturbance has also been shown in humans with the S(-) form. Studies in sheep have shown a higher threshold for convulsions with the S(-) form. These safer features are not at the expense of efficacy.

PHYSIOLOGY
Nephron

How does the nephron work?
The nephron consists of an individual renal tubule and its glomerulus. The tubule is divided into the following segments: proximal convoluted tubule, loop of Henle, distal tubule and collecting tubule.

Glomerulus: a network of capillaries invaginated into the dilated blind end of the nephron (Bowman's capsule). Blood enters the glomerulus from the afferent arteriole and leaves through the narrower efferent arteriole. The process of glomerular filtration allows the passage of an ultrafiltrate of plasma through the glomerular capillaries into Bowman's space and into the proximal tubule.

Proximal tubule: (a bulk reabsorber), responsible for the absorption of approximately 70% of the filtered sodium and water. Other substances such as chloride, calcium, bicarbonate, magnesium, glucose, phosphate and amino acids are reabsorbed here to a large extent. The reabsorption is isosmotic so the osmolality remains the same at the end of the proximal tubule (290 mosmol/kg). The rest of the tubule is the fine regulator.

Loop of Henle: consists of a thin descending limb which descends from the cortex into the medulla and an ascending limb which is thin at its lower end and becomes the thick ascending limb as it ascends back into the cortex. The loop of Henle reabsorbs 15–20% of the filtered sodium load. Chloride ions, water, magnesium, potassium and calcium are also reabsorbed. The countercurrent multiplier system operates in the loop of Henle. This is provided by the U-shaped arrangement of the peritubular capillaries (vasa recta) to the loop of Henle. The interstitial fluid osmolarity increases from isosmotic at the corticomedullary junction to 1200–1600 mosmol/l deep in the medulla. This gradient enables the fluid in the collecting tubules to be concentrated as the tubules run through the medulla, and urine which is hypertonic to plasma to be excreted. The most distal part of the loop of Henle is the macula densa, which is in contact with the afferent arteriole of its own glomerulus forming the juxtaglomerular apparatus. This apparatus is responsible for renin secretion in response to sympathetic stimulation, changes in afferent arteriolar wall pressure and changes in chloride flow past the macula densa.

Distal tubule: receives hypotonic fluid from the loop of Henle. The early part is relatively impermeable to sodium and water and can therefore maintain the gradients generated by the loop of Henle. About 5% of the filtered water is reabsorbed here. The permeability of the distal part is determined by the circulating level of ADH. ADH increases the permeability of the tubule causing water to be reabsorbed into the bloodstream and this increases urine concentration. The distal tubule is impermeable to urea.

Collecting system: collects urine from several distal tubules and runs through the hyperosmotic medulla to drain into the renal pelvis and ureters. This is the main segment for regulated sodium reabsorption, potassium reabsorption or secretion, hydrogen ion secretion (aldosterone-regulated), and water reabsorption (ADH regulated).

Viva 2b

CLINICAL

What are the likely causes for his deterioration?
He may have suffered any one of the following:
- Simple pneumothorax
- Tension pneumothorax
- Haemothorax
- Fat embolus

The latter is particularly likely in view of the history of fracture of a long bone.

How would you manage him?
He should be given supplemental oxygen whilst obtaining a chest X-ray and arterial blood gas sample after careful clinical examination.

If he has a tension pneumothorax then the above investigations should be postponed until he has been stabilised.

If he has a tension pneumothorax then initially a wide bore intravenous cannula should be inserted in the second intercostal space in the midclavicular line on the side of the pneumothorax, followed by insertion of a chest drain.

Intravenous access should be secured and fluids given as appropriate.

This man is found to have suffered a fat embolus.
What investigations would you perform, what would they be likely to show and how would you manage him?
An arterial blood gas sample should be taken for analysis; it would be likely to show hypoxaemia and hypocarbia.

The chest X-ray may be normal or show diffuse interstitial shadowing.

Urinalysis may reveal the presence of fat droplets, as may the sputum.

Management is supportive and involves the administration of oxygen to correct hypoxaemia; intubation and ventilation may be required.

Early fixation of the femoral fracture will prevent further fat embolism.

PHYSICS
Rotameters

What is a rotameter?
A rotameter is a constant pressure, variable orifice device used to measure gas flow in the anaesthetic machine accurately.

What safety devices are employed in flowmeters?
Flowmeter control knobs are labelled and colour coded. Compared with the other control knobs, the oxygen control knob is larger, protrudes further from the flowmeter block and has a different shape. It is always on the left-hand side of the block in the UK. The torque needed to operate the control knobs meets a UK safety standard so that it is high enough to try to avoid accidental readjustment. Most modern flowmeters incorporate devices that make it impossible to deliver nitrous oxide without a safe concentration of oxygen e.g. by linking their control valves via a chain, or gears or using pneumatic mixing valves. Oxygen is the last gas to be delivered to the mixed gas flow, so that if a gas leak occurs

the chance of a hypoxic mixture being delivered to the patient is minimised.

Some flowmeters have a mechanical stop on the oxygen flowmeter control so that a minimum oxygen flow of 200 ml/min occurs even when the control knob is fully closed. Flowmeter tubes are calibrated individually for highest accuracy. Flow restricters are present downstream of the flowmeter to prevent back pressure being exerted on the flowmeter and producing inaccurate readings. Other designs have the flow controls on the outlet to work at an increased pressure of several bar to minimise the relatively small pressure changes at the outlet.

Anti-static materials are used in order to prevent the bobbin or ball sticking to the wall of the flowmeter causing inaccurate readings. There should be good exposure of the top of the glass tubes to avoid concealment of bobbins so that high flow rates of gases are not hidden. This is particularly relevant for nitrous oxide.

PRACTICE EXAMINATION 3

MULTIPLE CHOICE QUESTION PAPER 3

90 Questions: time allowed 3 hours.
Indicate your answers with a tick or cross in the spaces provided.

3.1   The following antibiotics act by inhibiting cell wall synthesis:

❑ A cephalosporins
❑ B tetracyclines
❑ C aminoglycosides
❑ D penicillins
❑ E sulphonamides

3.2   L-dopa

❑ A is a metabolic product of dopamine
❑ B penetrates the CNS poorly
❑ C is not metabolised in peripheral tissues
❑ D can cause nausea
❑ E can cause arrhythmias

3.3   Propofol

❑ A is formulated in propylene glycol
❑ B has a pH greater than 10
❑ C is conjugated to glucuronides and sulphates in the liver
❑ D causes coronary vasodilatation
❑ E has a low hepatic clearance

3.4   The effects of α_2 adrenoreceptor agonists include

❑ A sedation
❑ B a dry mouth
❑ C cold extremities
❑ D bradycardia
❑ E reduced analgesic requirements

3.5   Drugs may produce hypotension by an action on

❑   A   parasympathetic ganglia
❑   B   α adrenoreceptors
❑   C   β adrenoreceptors
❑   D   noradrenaline synthesis
❑   E   noradrenaline release

3.6   Tricyclic antidepressants

❑   A   inhibit neuronal uptake of noradrenaline
❑   B   have a rapid onset of action
❑   C   may cause a dry mouth and constipation
❑   D   do not produce postural hypotension
❑   E   may produce tachycardia and palpitations

3.7   Ketamine

❑   A   is a racemic mixture
❑   B   increases cardiac output
❑   C   has an action at NMDA controlled ion channels
❑   D   induces anaesthesia in one arm brain circulation time
❑   E   has active metabolites

3.8   The following are potassium sparing:

❑   A   frusemide
❑   B   amiloride
❑   C   triamterene
❑   D   acetazolamide
❑   E   spironolactone

3.9   β adrenoreceptor blocking drugs

❏ A   increase myocardial oxygen consumption
❏ B   may have partial agonist activity
❏ C   may have a quinidine like effect
❏ D   may reduce hepatic blood flow
❏ E   reduce maximal exercise capacity

3.10   The blood-brain barrier is readily crossed by

❏ A   glycopyrrolate
❏ B   hyoscine
❏ C   neostigmine
❏ D   D-tubocurarine
❏ E   morphine

3.11   Diazepam

❏ A   has a longer terminal half-life in the elderly
❏ B   is metabolised to midazolam
❏ C   acts in the same time as thiopentone
❏ D   increases GABA concentrations in the brain
❏ E   is well absorbed following intramuscular injection

3.12   With regard to pharmacokinetics

❏ A   zero order kinetics indicates metabolism at a constant rate
❏ B   first order kinetics can change to zero order kinetics
❏ C   a three compartment model is a feature of fat soluble drugs
❏ D   drugs with large volumes of distribution have long half-lives
❏ E   compartments refer to anatomical structures

3.13 In severe liver disease

❏ A tubocurarine is potentiated
❏ B suxamethonium is potentiated
❏ C gallamine is potentiated
❏ D neostigmine is ineffective
❏ E atracurium is unaffected

3.14 The following drugs are more than 50% protein bound:

❏ A phenytoin
❏ B morphine
❏ C diazepam
❏ D atracurium
❏ E alfentanil

3.15 The following dilate the pupil:

❏ A neostigmine
❏ B cocaine
❏ C ganglion blockers
❏ D atenolol
❏ E codeine

3.16 The following are metabolised by cholinesterase:

❏ A procaine
❏ B neostigmine
❏ C mivacurium
❏ D suxamethonium
❏ E diamorphine

3.17   The following show zero order kinetics at normal doses:

- ❑   A   phenytoin
- ❑   B   morphine
- ❑   C   aspirin
- ❑   D   ethyl alcohol
- ❑   E   warfarin

3.18   Sodium nitroprusside

- ❑   A   acts via nitric oxide
- ❑   B   causes tachycardia
- ❑   C   should be protected from light
- ❑   D   lowers intracranial pressure
- ❑   E   increases pulmonary artery pressure

3.19   The clearance of a drug

- ❑   A   represents the removal of a given amount of drug in unit time
- ❑   B   represents the rate of elimination per unit concentration in blood
- ❑   C   equals the volume of distribution multiplied by the half-life
- ❑   D   equals the volume of distribution multiplied by a constant
- ❑   E   is inversely proportional to the half-life

3.20   The following have an elimination half-life of more than 24 hours:

- ❑   A   diazepam
- ❑   B   amiodarone
- ❑   C   chlorpropamide
- ❑   D   digoxin
- ❑   E   thiopentone

3.21 Coronary blood flow

- ❏ A   in health is affected by small (< 20 mmHg) changes in mean arterial BP
- ❏ B   is equal to diastolic blood pressure
- ❏ C   is mainly under humoral control
- ❏ D   increases following beta blockade by a direct vasodilator effect
- ❏ E   return is above 85% to the right atrium via the coronary sinus

3.22 In starvation

- ❏ A   muscle glycogen and brain glycogen are replenished by gluconeogenesis
- ❏ B   ketone bodies produced in the liver from free fatty acids can be utilised by brain cells, but glucose is still essential
- ❏ C   FFA oxidation in liver, muscle and heart is increased
- ❏ D   there is a fall in body potassium
- ❏ E   secondary to vomiting in children, the odour of breath is due to ketosis

3.23 The rate at which the alveolar concentration of an anaesthetic agent approaches the inspired concentration is a function of

- ❏ A   alveolar ventilation
- ❏ B   water solubility
- ❏ C   cardiac output
- ❏ D   saturated vapour pressure
- ❏ E   inspired concentration

3.24 In metabolic acidosis

- ❏ A   base excess is positive
- ❏ B   plasma bicarbonate never exceeds 30 mEq/l
- ❏ C   standard bicarbonate falls
- ❏ D $PaCO_2$ may be normal
- ❏ E   urine pH falls

3.25   The following are features of an active transport system:

❏   A   expenditure of energy
❏   B   independent of temperature
❏   C   unaffected by hypoxia
❏   D   movement against a concentration gradient
❏   E   maximal transport rate

3.26   Iron

❏   A   absorption is dependent on erythropoietin
❏   B   absorption is dependent on total body iron
❏   C   is carried in the plasma as transferrin
❏   D   absorption requires an intact colonic mucosa
❏   E   accumulation can result in a raised blood glucose

3.27   In a subject lying on his side breathing quietly

❏   A   blood flow is greater in the lower lung
❏   B   ventilation is greater in the lower lung
❏   C   V/Q is greater in blood coming from the lower lung
❏   D PaO_2 is greater in blood coming from the lower lung
❏   E $PaCO_2$ is greater in blood coming from the lower lung

3.28   On changing from standing to supine

❏   A   heart rate increases
❏   B   pressure in the leg veins increases
❏   C   capacitance of the pulmonary veins increases
❏   D   baroreceptor activity increases
❏   E   there is a diuresis

3.29 **The following are neurotransmitters at autonomic ganglia:**

❏ A histamine
❏ B bradykinin
❏ C adrenaline
❏ D methacholine
❏ E dopamine

3.30 **During quiet inspiration**

❏ A alveolar volume increases by 30%
❏ B abdominal muscles are active
❏ C sacrospinalis muscles are active
❏ D intrathoracic pressure decreases by a few mmHg
❏ E the ribcage does not move

3.31 **Immediately after transection of the spinal cord in the cervical region the following are seen:**

❏ A loss of bladder reflexes
❏ B hypotension
❏ C loss of the knee reflex
❏ D spastic paralysis
❏ E loss of sensation in the legs

3.32 **The sensation of pain**

❏ A is conveyed mainly in the dorsal column
❏ B is augmented by beta endorphin
❏ C can be modified by cutting the spinothalamic tract
❏ D can be modified by strenuous exercise
❏ E can be modified by non painful stimuli of the same area

3.33   Increased gamma motor neurone activity will result in

- ❏   A   skeletal muscle relaxation
- ❏   B   uterine contraction
- ❏   C   vasodilatation
- ❏   D   increased tone of voluntary muscles
- ❏   E   hyperactive tendon reflexes

3.34   Concerning fetal circulation

- ❏   A   it is possible for vena caval blood to reach the aorta without going through the left ventricle or left atrium
- ❏   B   the PaO_2 in the descending aorta is less than in the ductus arteriosus
- ❏   C   foramen ovale closes at birth because of the increased left atrial pressure
- ❏   D   flow in the ductus arteriosus stops/reverses at birth because of decreased pulmonary vascular resistance
- ❏   E   highly oxygenated blood reaches the head of the fetus via the right ventricle

3.35   The following influence aldosterone:

- ❏   A   surgical stress
- ❏   B   high sodium intake
- ❏   C   renal ischaemia
- ❏   D   angiotensin
- ❏   E   plasma potassium concentration

3.36   The physiological response to haemorrhagic shock consists of

- ❏   A   increased sympathetic activity
- ❏   B   production of renin
- ❏   C   increased production of erythropoietin
- ❏   D   increased baroreceptor activity
- ❏   E   increased chemoreceptor activity

3.37 In the Valsalva manoeuvre there is

❑ A an initial rise in blood pressure
❑ B an initial tachycardia followed by bradycardia
❑ C a fall in cardiac output
❑ D an increase in renal blood flow
❑ E an abnormal response in diabetics

3.38 Potassium

❑ A excretion is increased by aldosterone
❑ B normal excretion is up to 100 mmol/day
❑ C excretion is decreased for up to 2 to 3 days postoperatively
❑ D is filtered by the glomerulus
❑ E is actively absorbed in the proximal tubule and loop of Henle

3.39 The intrinsic clotting cascade is associated with

❑ A factor IX
❑ B factor VII
❑ C a faster speed of action than the extrinsic system
❑ D initial activation of factor VIII
❑ E an enzyme cascade

3.40 Cerebrospinal fluid (CSF)

❑ A volume is 20% of intracranial volume
❑ B pressure pulsates with blood pressure and respiration
❑ C production is 0.4 mg/min from the choroid plexus
❑ D is absorbed from the arachnoid villi
❑ E pressure follows cerebral blood flow in the short term

3.41 **The following can be used for the measurement of temperature:**

❏ A the Seebeck effect
❏ B alcohol thermometers
❏ C mercury thermometers
❏ D resistance
❏ E interferometer

3.42 **Concerning the sterilisation of anaesthetic equipment**

❏ A boiling in water for 15 mins at atmospheric pressure kills bacteria and spores
❏ B an autoclave pressure of 1 bar at a temperature of 120°C for 15 minutes will kill all living organisms
❏ C ethylene oxide is only bactericidal
❏ D ethylene oxide takes 2–4 hours to be completely effective
❏ E a 0.1% solution of chlorhexidine will sterilise an endotracheal tube in 3 minutes

3.43 **Minimum alveolar concentration (MAC)**

❏ A is an index of potency of intravenous anaesthetics
❏ B is measured in volumes %
❏ C can be determined by probit analysis
❏ D is affected by age
❏ E is a correlate of oil/water solubility

3.44 **Measurement of airway resistance may entail the use of**

❏ A oesophageal balloon
❏ B body plethysmography
❏ C pneumotachograph
❏ D stethograph
❏ E Haldane alveolar tube

3.45 Basal metabolic rate

- ❑ A is 70 kJ/m²/hour
- ❑ B may be measured using an ergometer
- ❑ C is high in tropical climates
- ❑ D is low in children
- ❑ E is always elevated in patients with a goitre

3.46 Plasma volume can be measured using

- ❑ A para-amino hippuric acid
- ❑ B inulin
- ❑ C radioactively labelled albumin
- ❑ D Evans' blue
- ❑ E creatinine

3.47 Oxygen rotameters

- ❑ A can be used with nitrous oxide
- ❑ B consist of a bulb in a cylinder
- ❑ C are affected by back pressure
- ❑ D have a linear scale
- ❑ E are an example of a variable orifice flowmeter

3.48 Pressure can be expressed as

- ❑ A force per unit area
- ❑ B kg/m/s²
- ❑ C Pascals
- ❑ D Newton/m²
- ❑ E bars

3.49   A paramagnetic gas analyser is useful for the measurement of

- ❏   A   halothane
- ❏   B   oxygen
- ❏   C   nitrogen
- ❏   D   nitrous oxide
- ❏   E   carbon dioxide

3.50   Resistance to current flow in a wire changes with

- ❏   A   tension in the wire
- ❏   B   temperature in the wire
- ❏   C   length of the wire
- ❏   D   diameter of the wire
- ❏   E   changes in a semiconductor

3.51   Viscosity

- ❏   A   decreases as the temperature of a gas increases
- ❏   B   of a liquid rises as its temperature rises
- ❏   C   is dependent on molecular cohesiveness
- ❏   D   is dependent on Van der Waal's forces
- ❏   E   of oxygen/helium mixtures is less than that of oxygen/nitrous oxide mixtures

3.52   Surface tension

- ❏   A   changes with temperature
- ❏   B   can be measured in pascal metres
- ❏   C   is due to molecular cohesion
- ❏   D   leads to a mercury manometer over-reading
- ❏   E   depends on viscosity

3.53 **According to Boyle's law**

❏ A PV = k
❏ B 1 gram mol occupies 22.4 litres at room temperature
❏ C a plot of P versus V is a straight line
❏ D a plot of P versus V is a rectangular hyperbole
❏ E a plot of V versus P gives a reciprocal of k

3.54 **The following disadvantages apply to these methods of temperature measurement:**

❏ A mercury in a glass thermometer has a slow response time
❏ B platinum resistance thermometer probes are not interchangeable
❏ C platinum resistance thermometer probes have a slow response time
❏ D thermistors can become unstable over a period of a few months
❏ E thermocouples have so many disadvantages that they are not in clinical use

3.55 **Gas or air can be satisfactorily humidified in the following ways:**

❏ A passage through the upper respiratory tract
❏ B passage through a cold water bath
❏ C using the Bernoulli effect
❏ D using heated water humidifiers
❏ E using the Joule Thompson effect

3.56 **The following are properties of nitrous oxide:**

❏ A a boiling point of −8°C
❏ B nitrous oxide cylinders have a filling ratio of 0.9
❏ C helium and nitrous oxide can be used in the same flowmeter
❏ D a MAC value greater than 100%
❏ E a critical temperature of 36.5°C

3.57   In the measurement of CVP

❏   A   the catheter must be less than 20 cm long
❏   B   the ideal catheter diameter is greater than 0.25 cm
❏   C   the reference point must be the angle of Louis
❏   D   the patient must be lying flat
❏   E   the ventilator should be disconnected when taking the CVP
            reading

3.58   The amount of gas that will dissolve in a liquid is determined by

❏   A   temperature
❏   B   ambient pressure
❏   C   liquid
❏   D   gas/liquid coefficient
❏   E   molecular weight of the gas but not of the liquid

3.59   Spirometry can be used to measure

❏   A   functional residual capacity (FRC)
❏   B   total lung capacity (TLC)
❏   C   residual volume (RV)
❏   D   expiratory reserve volume
❏   E   functional inspiratory reserve volume

**3.60   Concerning the location of vaporisers within the anaesthetic
            circuit**

❏   A   with the vaporiser inside a circle (VIC), the inflow gas contains
            an unknown concentration of volatile agent
❏   B   with VIC, an accurate vaporiser, efficient at low flows, should
            be used to maintain an accurate vapour flow within the circuit
❏   C   with the vaporiser outside the circle (VOC) an inefficient
            vaporiser is adequate because inspired concentrations are not
            critical
❏   D   with VOC, the anaesthetic vapour concentration within the
            circuit is dependent upon uptake
❏   E   with VIC and low fresh gas flow, the inspired concentration is
            greater than the vaporiser setting

3.61 The following are equivalent to a pressure of one atmosphere:

- ❑ A 100 mmHg
- ❑ B 1000 cmH$_2$O
- ❑ C 760 bar
- ❑ D 12 torr
- ❑ E 10 kPa

3.62 An intra-aortic balloon pump will increase

- ❑ A heart rate
- ❑ B myocardial workload
- ❑ C coronary perfusion pressure
- ❑ D left ventricular work
- ❑ E left ventricular afterload

3.63 Concerning pacemakers and anaesthesia

- ❑ A a magnet placed over a demand pacemaker will convert it to a fixed rate pacemaker
- ❑ B unipolar diathermy should be used
- ❑ C a patient with a pacemaker may safely enter an MRI scanner
- ❑ D post-operative shivering may affect pacemaker function
- ❑ E induction of anaesthesia may alter pacemaker function

3.64 Entonox

- ❑ A is stored in cylinders at 137 bar
- ❑ B has a critical temperature of –7°C
- ❑ C can be administered by registered midwives
- ❑ D can lead to megaloblastic anaemia after prolonged exposure
- ❑ E is a 50:50 mixture of nitric oxide and oxygen

3.65   With regard to Tuohy needles and epidural catheters

❏   A   the filter has pores of 22 microns diameter
❏   B   the standard needle is 16 gauge
❏   C   the needle is 10 cm long
❏   D   hanging drop technique may be used to locate the epidural space
❏   E   Lee markings are present at 1 cm intervals on the Tuohy needle

3.66   In an exponential process

❏   A   37% of the process is completed in one time constant
❏   B   95% of the process is completed in three time constants
❏   C   the rate of change is constant
❏   D   washout curves are exponential processes
❏   E   time constant and half-life are synonymous

3.67   Helium

❏   A   is stored as a liquid
❏   B   is a useful treatment for bronchospasm
❏   C   has similar viscosity to oxygen
❏   D   supports combustion
❏   E   is a narcotic at pressure

3.68   Wright's respirometer

❏   A   is inaccurate at flows of < 1 l/min
❏   B   is a turbine
❏   C   is affected by viscosity of gas
❏   D   is affected by humidity
❏   E   can be used to measure peak flow

3.69   Peak flow

- ❑   A   is not effort dependent
- ❑   B   is measured by the pneumotachograph
- ❑   C   is measured by the vitalograph
- ❑   D   is reduced in acute asthma
- ❑   E   has a diurnal variation

3.70   The Severinghaus electrode

- ❑   A   consists of CO_2 sensitive glass
- ❑   B   is better with gases than with blood
- ❑   C   measures pH
- ❑   D   is affected by nitrous oxide
- ❑   E   contains bicarbonate ions in the electrolyte solution

3.71   Soda lime

- ❑   A   contains 70% calcium hydroxide and 30% sodium hydroxide
- ❑   B   may not be used with desflurane
- ❑   C   may warm to 60°C during active CO_2 absorption
- ❑   D   use has been associated with methaemoglobinaemia
- ❑   E   produces humidification of inspired gases

3.72   An arterial line in the radial artery can lead to

- ❑   A   fatal haemorrhage
- ❑   B   pulmonary embolism
- ❑   C   intracerebral embolism
- ❑   D   paraesthesia at the base of the thumb
- ❑   E   septicaemia

3.73   The thromboelastograph (TEG)

❑ A   will be a flat line if a heparinised sample is used
❑ B   provides information about platelet function
❑ C   provides information about thrombolysis
❑ D   can be used to determine what blood products a bleeding
         patient may require
❑ E   is much slower than laboratory estimation of PT, APTT and
         platelet count

3.74   Transoesophageal echo (TOE)

❑ A   can be used to assess cardiac output
❑ B   employs ultrasound
❑ C   is a very sensitive detector of pulmonary emboli
❑ D   cannot be used with diathermy
❑ E   is a Doppler probe

3.75   The hazard of microshock can be reduced by the use of

❑ A   saline filled intracardiac catheters
❑ B   large area diathermy plates
❑ C   battery powered appliances
❑ D   multiple earth paths
❑ E   isolated (floating) power supply

3.76   Halothane vapour

❑ A   concentration can be measured using a refractometer
❑ B   is less dense than nitrous oxide
❑ C   will absorb ultraviolet radiation
❑ D   can be measured by infrared absorption
❑ E   can be measured by changes in the elasticity of silicone
         rubber

3.77   Concerning the Mapleson classification of breathing systems

❑   A   the Bain system is a Mapleson D system
❑   B   all the systems are partial rebreathing systems
❑   C   there are no valves in the Mapleson E system
❑   D   the Mapleson A system is the most efficient for spontaneous ventilation
❑   E   Humphrey designed a system incorporating the A, D and E systems into one breathing system

3.78   Nitrous oxide cylinders

❑   A   are made of molybdenum steel
❑   B   have a filling ratio of 0.67
❑   C   the cylinder pressure is 137 bar
❑   D   the cylinder pressure falls linearly with use
❑   E   have a pin index number of 3,6

3.79   The following are SI units:

❑   A   pascal
❑   B   hertz
❑   C   pounds per square inch
❑   D   watt
❑   E   joule

3.80   Cricoid presssure

❑   A   was first described by Sellick
❑   B   requires the application of a force of 440 Newtons
❑   C   is performed to prevent vomitus from entering the bronchial tree
❑   D   must be applied at extubation as well as intubation
❑   E   may make visualisation of the vocal cords more difficult

3.81 Pulse oximeters

- ❑ A may cause burns to the skin under the probe
- ❑ B are inaccurate in patients with pigmented skin
- ❑ C are inaccurate in the presence of haemoglobin F
- ❑ D are inaccurate in the presence of methaemoglobin
- ❑ E have a slower response time than transcutaneous oxygen electrodes

3.82 Regarding anaesthetic equipment

- ❑ A a 14G cannula can deliver a maximal flow rate of 280 ml/min
- ❑ B a standard blood giving set has a filter of 150 microns diameter
- ❑ C disposable endotracheal tubes are implant tested on mice
- ❑ D the Fraser–Sweatman filling device for isoflurane is green
- ❑ E the LMA should only be re-used 14 times

3.83 Regarding the gas laws

- ❑ A Boyle's law states that at constant pressure the volume of a fixed mass of gas is inversely related to its temperature
- ❑ B Avogadro's hypothesis states that the molar mass of a gas occupies 222.4 litres
- ❑ C Charles' law states that at constant temperature the volume of a fixed mass of gas is inversely related to its pressure
- ❑ D $PV = kT$
- ❑ E they all apply only to a gas at standard temperature and pressure

3.84 The Hageni-Poiseuille law states that, assuming laminar flow

- ❑ A the flow of liquid along a tube is inversely related to its length
- ❑ B the flow is doubled for every doubling in diameter of the tube
- ❑ C viscosity is not important
- ❑ D density is not important
- ❑ E the law only applies to Newtonian liquids

3.85   Capnography

❏ A   depends upon absorption of infrared light
❏ B   depends upon the presence of two or more different atoms in the molecule being measured
❏ C   the absorption spectra for carbon dioxide and nitrous oxide are widely separated
❏ D   may be inaccurate with very rapid respiratory rates
❏ E   reliably confirms correct placement of the endotracheal tube

3.86   Oxygen can be measured by

❏ A   paramagnetic analyser
❏ B   capnography
❏ C   a fuel cell
❏ D   cathode ray oscilloscope
❏ E   pulse oximetry

3.87   Concerning the Mapleson E breathing system (Ayre's T-piece)

❏ A   during spontaneous ventilation the fresh gas flow should be 2.5–3 x the patient's minute volume
❏ B   the volume of the corrugated tube must exceed the patient's tidal volume
❏ C   Jackson-Rees modified the system by adding a closed bag to the end of the corrugated tube
❏ D   scavenging from the Mapleson F system can be done easily
❏ E   it should be used in children < 30 kg

3.88   The critical temperature

❏ A   is the temperature above which that substance cannot be liquefied by pressure
❏ B   of oxygen is –118°C
❏ C   of nitrous oxide is 36.5°C
❏ D   of Entonox is –6°C
❏ E   is the temperature below which that substance exists as liquid and vapour

3.89   The following are the correct pin-index numbers:

❑   A   oxygen 2, 5
❑   B   cyclopropane 3, 6
❑   C   nitrous oxide 3, 5
❑   D   helium 6, 7
❑   E   entonox no pin index

3.90   Nitrous oxide

❑   A   supports combustion
❑   B   was discovered by Joseph Priestley
❑   C   is supplied from pipelines at a pressure of 4 bar
❑   D   has a MAC of 1.05%
❑   E   Gardner Quincy Colton first used it as an anaesthetic in 1844
          to assist the extraction of a tooth from Mr Horace Wells

PRACTICE EXAM 3: OSCE PAPER 3

16 Stations: time allowed approximately 2 hours.

STATION 3.1

You are called to the Accident & Emergency Department to see a 13-year-old boy who has a pyrexia of 39°C, headache and a non-blanching rash over his abdomen.

(a) What is the diagnosis?

(b) What other immediate investigations are necessary?

(c) What is the management?

STATION 3.2

A lady of 45 is brought to the Accident and Emergency Department by her husband, having taken a large number of paracetamol tablets 48 hours earlier. She is obviously jaundiced, but otherwise appears well.

Investigations reveal

INR	6.0	Sodium	130	Potassium	4.5
AST	3,400	Glucose	1.8		

(a) What is the diagnosis?

(b) Explain the blood results.

(c) Where should this lady be managed?

(d) What important initial management should be undertaken?

STATION 3.3

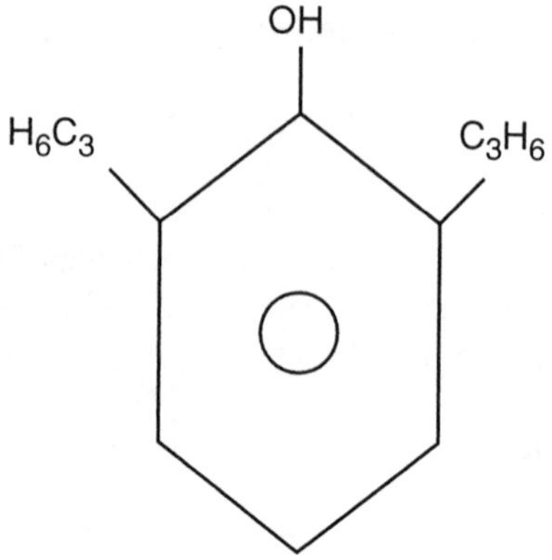

OH

H_6C_3 C_3H_6

Fig. 3.3

(a) What is this?

(b) What are the main side-effects of this compound?

STATION 3.4

Blood results

Na 130	pH 7.23	Hb 14.7
K 6.4	PaCO$_2$ 4.19	WCC 16.3 (Neutr 13.5)
Urea 12.9	PaO$_2$ 13.36	Plt 2.64
Creat 128	HCO$_3^-$ 14.7	
Glucose 67	BE -9.6	

(a) What is your diagnosis?

(b) How should this be managed?

(c) What are possible triggers for this problem?

(d) What types of diabetics are more likely to get this?

STATION 3.5

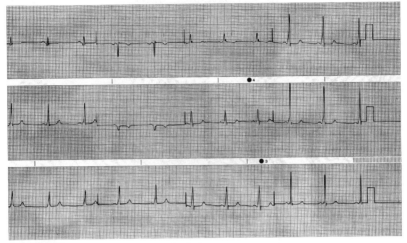

Exercise III, Patient 14

Fig. 3.5

(a) What does this ECG show?

(b) What is the danger of anaesthesia?

(c) What should be done prior to anaesthesia?

STATION 3.6

How would you examine and assess a 65-year-old man who is awaiting elective surgery for a hernia repair and is known to have ischaemic heart disease?

STATION 3.7

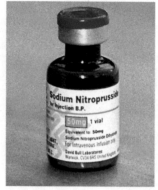

Fig. 3.7

(a) What agent is contained in this vial?

(b) What storage precautions are necessary?

(c) Why?

(d) What is the main clinical indication for this agent?

(e) How is it reconstituted for use?

(f) How should it be kept during use?

(g) What is the dosage?

(h) What is the maximal dosage?

(i) What dangers are there with prolonged use?

(j) Manage sodium nitroprusside toxicity.

STATION 3.8

Please state whether the following statements regarding the ECG shown below are **True** or **False**.

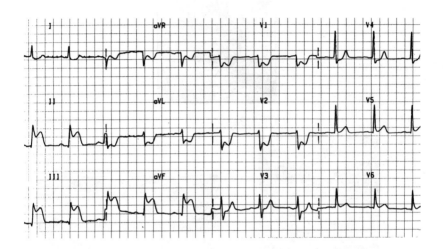

Fig. 3.8

	True	False
(a) The axis is normal	❑	❑
(b) There is evidence of pericarditis	❑	❑
(c) The patient should be given thrombolytic therapy	❑	❑
(d) The patient is at increased risk of complete heart block	❑	❑

STATION 3.9

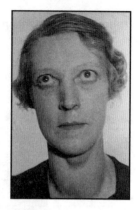

Fig.3.9a

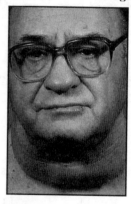

Fig. 3.9b

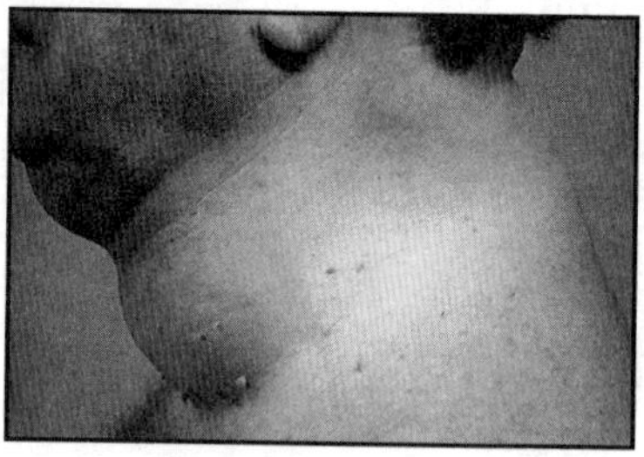

Fig.3.9c

1. *Figure 3.9a*
(a) What condition does this lady suffer from?

(b) What needs to be done before she is fit for routine elective surgery?

(c) What might you expect to find on clinical examination of this lady?

2. *Figures 3.9b and 3.9c*
(a) From what condition does the man suffer?

(b) What problems might one expect to find on clinical examination?

(c) He is booked for partial thyroidectomy. What are the relevant anaesthetic implications?

(d) If he developed respiratory obstruction post-operatively what might be the likely causes?

STATION 3.10

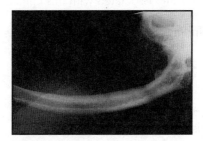

Fig. 3.10

(a) What is the diagnosis?

(b) What complications can arise in this disease and what is the relevance to anaesthesia?

STATION 3.11

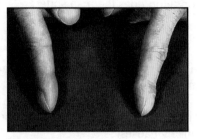

Fig. 3.11

(a) What does this slide show?

(b) What conditions are associated with this clinical sign?

(c) How might finding this clinical sign affect anaesthesia?

STATION 3.12

You are asked to give a general anaesthetic to a patient requiring electroconvulsive therapy (ECT).

(a) What are the physiological consequences of ECT?

(b) What are the contraindications to ECT?

STATION 3.13

An elderly lady has sustained a Colles' fracture. It has been decided she will have a Biers block.

An interested medical student asks you to explain what you are going to do; please do so.

STATION 3.14

(a) What is soda lime?

(b) Why are circle systems used?

STATION 3.15

How would you check your anaesthetic machine before starting the first list of the day?

STATION 3.16

Communication

Explain an epidural versus a spinal versus a combined spinal epidural (CSE) to a patient who is awaiting surgery to his lower limb, but does not want a general anaesthetic.

Viva 3a

PHARMACOLOGY
Anti-emetics

What neurotransmitters are involved in nausea and vomiting? Where would we encounter them?

Classify anti-emetics by their mechanism of action. Where are their main sites of action?

How can we administer anti-emetics?

Do you know of any drugs that can be administered transdermally?

PHYSIOLOGY
Gastric motility

What factors control gastric emptying?

What would therefore promote gastric stasis?

Describe the vomiting act.

Viva 3b

CLINICAL

A 40-year-old male patient is brought to the Accident and Emergency Department in status epilepticus.
You are asked to assess him by the Accident and Emergency SHO.

What is your initial management?

What are the common causes of seizures?

PHYSICS
Defibrillators

What is a defibrillator? How does it work?

What types of defibrillators are generally available? What are their advantages and disadvantages?

Why are our first two shocks only 200 Joules in the ventricular fibrillation/ventricular tachycardia (VF/VT) guidelines?

3.1   **Answers: A D**

The penicillins are bactericidal and act by inhibiting cell wall synthesis. Their principal side-effect is a hypersensitivity rash. The cephalosporins are bactericidal and interfere with the final stage of bacterial cell wall synthesis. Like the penicillins the principal side-effect of cephalosporins is a hypersensitivity rash. 10% of patients with penicillin hypersensitivity will also be allergic to a cephalosporin. The aminoglycosides act by binding to bacterial ribosomes leading to misreading of mRNA. The aminoglycosides are potentially ototoxic and nephrotoxic. Sulphonamides act as competitive antagonists of folic acid which certain bacteria require. Tetracyclines, like the aminoglycosides bind to bacterial ribosomes.

3.2   **Answers: D E**

L-dopa is the precursor of dopamine. L-dopa crosses the blood-brain barrier but dopamine does not. L-dopa is converted peripherally by the enzyme dopa decarboxylase to dopamine. Patients are usually given, in addition to L-dopa, an L-dopa decarboxylase inhibitor to prevent this conversion as dopamine may cause arrhythmias or nausea.

3.3   **Answer: C**

Propofol is formulated in a white emulsion containing purified egg phosphatide, glycerol and soya bean oil. The pH of propofol is 10. Propofol is metabolised mainly in the liver and conjugated to inactive products which are then excreted in the urine. Total body clearance is 1.5–2 litres/min. Although propofol causes peripheral vasodilatation it has little effect on the coronary vasculature.

3.4   **Answers: A B C D E**

Alpha 2 adrenoreceptor agonists, such as clonidine, act to reduce sympathetic outflow from the central nervous system. This results in bradycardia and hypotension. In addition these drugs are sedative and analgesic and reduce the requirement for other anaesthetic agents. They also cause a dry mouth and may cause Raynaud's phenomenon.

3.5   **Answers: B C D E**

The answer to this question lies in the two equations:

1. Blood pressure (BP) = Cardiac output (CO) X Total peripheral
resistance (TPR)

and

2. CO = Stroke volume(SV) X Heart rate (HR).

TPR is controlled by vasoconstriction, produced by stimulation of
α 1 adrenoreceptors. These receptors are stimulated by the
neurotransmitter noradrenaline released from nerve terminals.
Block of β receptors will cause a fall in heart rate and stroke volume
thus leading to hypotension.

3.6   **Answers: A C E**

Tricyclic antidepressants act by inhibiting the re-uptake of
noradrenaline into nerve terminals. In addition they have
anticholinergic effects and this is why they are often associated with
tachycardia, palpitations and arrhythmias, as well as dry mouth and
constipation. Their onset of action may take several weeks, whilst
the unwanted side-effects may occur much earlier.

3.7   **Answers: A B C E**

Ketamine is a phencyclidine derivative which acts at NMDA
receptors. It is a racemic mixture; the +enantiomer being responsible for the useful effects such as analgesia; the – enantiomer being
responsible for the side-effects. It is a sympathomimetic agent
causing tachycardia, increased cardiac output and hypertension. It
acts very slowly compared with other anaesthetic agents and it has
active metabolites, such as nor-ketamine.

3.8   **Answers: B C E**

Most thiazide and loop diuretics lead to hypokalaemia. Amiloride
and triamterene are potassium sparing diuretics. Acetazolamide is a
carbonic anhydrase inhibitor. Spironolactone is an aldosterone
antagonist, and therefore is potassium sparing.

3.9   **Answers: B C**

Beta blockers are negatively chronotropic and inotropic. Thus they reduce myocardial oxygen consumption and increase maximal exercise capacity. Some beta blockers are partial agonists and some have quinidine like membrane stabilising effects. Whilst beta blockers may cause peripheral vasoconstriction, they have no effect on hepatic blood flow.

3.10   **Answers: B E**

Drugs which are highly ionised cannot cross the blood–brain barrier, whilst lipid soluble drugs can. Equally drugs which are highly protein bound or of a large molecular weight do not cross readily. All of the anticholinesterases, except physostigmine, are highly ionised quaternary amines and therefore do not cross the blood–brain barrier. Hyoscine and atropine are both tertiary amines, less ionised, and thus able to cross. Glycopyrrolate is a quaternary amine. Morphine crosses the barrier because of its very high lipid solubility.

3.11   **Answers: A D**

Diazepam, as a benzodiazepine, acts within the central nervous system by stimulating inhibitory gamma aminobutyric acid receptors (GABA type A receptors). Onset of action is slower than thiopentone whilst the elimination half-life is prolonged, due mainly to the production of active metabolites such as temazepam, oxazepam and N-desmethyldiazepam, which has an elimination half-life of between 40 and 200 hours!

3.12

Answers: A B C D

Pharmacokinetics, the absorption, distribution, metabolism and excretion of drugs, may be described as what the body does to the drug. Pharmacodynamics, pharmacological effects at receptor level, may be described as what the drug does to the body. In zero order kinetics a constant amount of drug is metabolised per unit of time. This applies to alcohol which is metabolised by the enzyme alcohol dehydrogenase. In first order kinetics a constant percentage of drug is metabolised per unit of time. It is possible for kinetics to change from first to zero order, as can happen with phenytoin, for example. The volume of distribution (Vd) is the apparent volume into which the drug is spread and depends on fat solubility to a large extent. Drugs with a large Vd tend to be metabolised relatively slowly and so have long half-lives. Compartment models are used to describe the pharmacokinetics of drugs, although compartments do not refer to actual anatomical entities.

3.13

Answers: A B E

Tubocurarine, pancuronium and vecuronium are all partly excreted in bile and therefore in severe liver disease their action is potentiated. Gallamine is mainly excreted renally and its action is not significantly potentiated in liver disease. Atracurium is unique in that its metabolism and elimination is independent of either renal or liver function. It undergoes a pH dependent spontaneous process termed Hoffman degradation and alkaline ester hydrolysis. Suxamethonium is metabolised by plasma cholinesterase, concentrations of which are much reduced in severe liver disease. Neostigmine acts by competitively antagonising the action of the enzyme acetylcholinesterase, and it is unaffected by liver disease.

3.14

Answer: A

Phenytoin is extensively protein bound. Other anaesthetic drugs which are highly protein bound include the local anaesthetic agents and thiopentone.

3.15   **Answers: B C**

The size of the pupil is controlled by the autonomic nervous system. Parasympathetic stimulation causes miosis, whilst dilatation of the pupil is caused by sympathetic stimulation. Thus neostigmine, by inhibiting the breakdown of acetylcholine, is parasympathomimetic and causes miosis. Opiates, such as codeine, stimulate the Edinger–Westphal nucleus of the oculomotor nerve, which is a purely parasympathetic nerve. It is by this mechanism that they cause miosis. Atenolol acts as a competitive antagonist at beta adrenoreceptors. The pupil is innervated by alpha-1 receptors, so beta blockers have no effect on the size of the pupil. Cocaine inhibits the re-uptake of noradrenaline at nerve endings and this sympathomimetic effect causes pupillary dilatation. Ganglion blockers cause mydriasis.

3.16   **Answers: A C D**

Plasma cholinesterase is responsible for the metabolism of a number of drugs including suxamethonium, mivacurium and the ester group of local anaesthetic agents, of which procaine is one.

3.17   **Answer: D**

Zero order kinetics (saturation kinetics) occur when a drug is metabolised by an enzyme. This applies to alcohol which is metabolised by alcohol dehydrogenase. The quantity of alcohol metabolised per unit time is constant as the enzyme system is saturatable. Although phenytoin may exhibit first and zero order kinetics, it only exhibits zero order kinetics in excessive doses.

3.18   **Answers: A B C**

Sodium nitroprusside (SNP) is a vasodilator which acts via conversion to nitric oxide. The solution, once prepared, is unstable and must therefore be protected from light. Reflex tachycardia is marked with SNP. SNP may lead to an increase in intracranial pressure due to dilatation of cerebral vessels. SNP will lower pulmonary artery pressure.

3.19   **Answers: A D E**

The clearance of a drug (Cl) is the volume of plasma that is cleared of the drug in unit time. Cl = Vd (volume of distribution) x k.

3.20   **Answers: A B C D E**

All of the drugs mentioned have a very long half-life. Diazepam has a half-life in excess of 200 hours due to its conversion to a number of active metabolites. Thiopentone undergoes metabolism according to zero order kinetics so that only 10–15% of the original dose of drug is eliminated every hour.

3.21   **Answers: All false**

The myocardium is supplied with oxygenated blood by the right and left coronary arteries. Venous drainage from the left ventricle passes via the coronary sinus to the right atrium.

Coronary blood flow occurs mainly in diastole and is therefore dependent upon diastolic blood pressure. In addition, as the length of diastole is dependent on heart rate, so is the coronary perfusion. As beta blockade slows heart rate it leads to improved myocardial blood flow. Coronary blood flow is determined primarily by myocardial oxygen demand. Small changes in blood pressure in the healthy person have little effect on coronary blood flow due to autoregulation in the vascular bed.

3.22   **Answers: B C D E**

In starvation, body glycogen stores are exhausted within 24–48 hours and subsequent energy must be obtained from other sources. Ketone bodies can be used by the brain but glucose is still essential. Hypokalaemia occurs and may be fatal.

3.23   **Answers: A C E**

The rate at which the alveolar concentration (FA) of an anaesthetic agent approaches the inspired concentration (FI) depends on:

- inspired concentration
- alveolar ventilation
- blood/gas solubility of the agent
- cardiac output

The alveolar concentration of the agent rises more rapidly as the alveolar ventilation increases. The relation with cardiac output is inverse. The alveolar concentration of an agent that is relatively insoluble in blood will rise more rapidly than that of a soluble agent. The rate at which FA approaches FI is directly related to the inspired concentration of the agent.

3.24   Answers: B C D E

Metabolic acidosis is characterised by a reduced pH, reduced plasma bicarbonate and a base deficit. The normal compensatory mechanism is hyperventilation and a reduction in $PaCO_2$, although the $PaCO_2$ may be normal.

The normal plasma bicarbonate is 22–30 mEq/l. In acidosis this is reduced.

3.25   Answers: A D E

Active transport is the movement of a substance across a membrane against a concentration gradient. This requires expenditure of energy and is therefore affected by hypoxia and temperature. Active transport systems are characterised by maximal transport rates.

3.26   Answers: B C E

Iron is absorbed in the small intestine and transported in the plasma as transferrin. Iron is stored as ferritin. The amount of iron absorbed is determined by the amount of ferritin and by total iron binding capacity. Iron overload, haemosiderosis, may cause glucose intolerance.

3.27   Answers: A B E

Although both ventilation and perfusion are greater in the lower lung, the increase in blood flow is greater than the increase in ventilation and thus the V/Q is less in blood coming from the lower lung. This means that blood from the lower lung has a lower PaO_2 and a higher $PaCO_2$.

3.28   Answer: C

On changing from standing to supine the heart rate falls and the blood pressure increases. As a result there is decreased baroreceptor activity.

3.29   Answers: All false

Acetylcholine is the neurotransmitter at all autonomic ganglia.

3.30   Answer: A

During quiet inspiration the diaphragm and intercostal muscles are active but the accessory muscles such as sacrospinalis are not used. Intrathoracic pressure decreases by 5–10 cmH_2O and alveolar volume increases by a third.

3.31   **Answers: B C E**

Immediately after transection of the spinal cord so called spinal shock occurs. This consists of hypotension due to loss of sympathetic tone, areflexia and loss of sensation below the level of cord transection.

3.32   **Answers: C D E**

Pain sensation is transmitted by fibres travelling in the spino-thalamic tracts. It is vibration and joint position sense that are conveyed in the dorsal columns. The endorphins are endogenous opioid-like substances which are analgesic. The sensation of pain can be modified by strenuous exercise or by non painful stimuli in the same area; this is how transcutaneous nerve stimulation (TENS) works.

3.33   **Answers: D E**

Gamma motor efferent fibres are found solely in striated skeletal muscle and are not present in the smooth muscle found in the uterus and vascular wall. Increased activity in these efferents leads to increased muscle tone and hyperreflexia.

3.34   **Answers: A C D**

The ductus arteriosus is a connection between the pulmonary artery and aorta which is patent in the neonate and closes shortly after birth when the pulmonary vascular resistance drops. The ductus carries blood which has entered the right heart from the superior vena cava. This blood then passes from the pulmonary artery to the descending aorta. The foramen ovale is another temporary connection in the foetal heart; in this case between the atria. At birth the rise in left atrial pressure and drop in pulmonary vascular resistance leads to closure of the foramen ovale, although 10% of adults have a functionally patent foramen ovale.

3.35   **Answers: A B C D E**

Aldosterone is a mineralocorticoid steroid hormone produced by the zona glomerulosa of the adrenal cortex. It acts on the distal tubule of the kidney, promoting sodium reabsorption in exchange for potassium and hydrogen ions. The production of aldosterone is controlled by the renin–angiotensin system. Renin is produced by the juxtaglomerular apparatus of the afferent arteriole of the glomerulus. Its secretion is increased in response to hypovolaemia, reduced renal blood flow and hyponatraemia. Renin acts on angiotensinogen, a plasma protein, converting it to angiotensin I, which in turn is converted to angiotensin II. Angiotensin II is an extremely potent vasoconstrictor and leads to the release of aldosterone. Aldosterone release is also stimulated by surgical stress, anxiety and haemorrhage. In addition hyponatraemia, hyperkalaemia and adrenocorticotrophic hormone (ACTH) all cause increased aldosterone release.

3.36   **Answers: A B C E**

Haemorrhage leads to increased sympathetic activity, with vasoconstriction and tachycardia. This helps to maintain cardiac output and keep vital organs such as the brain, kidneys and heart perfused. The reduced renal perfusion that results from haemorrhage activates the renin–angiotensin–aldosterone system and leads to increased release of antidiuretic hormone (ADH) from the posterior pituitary. This collective neurohumoral response leads to renal retention of sodium and water, restoring intravascular volume. In the longer term, haemorrhage will stimulate erythro-poietin production by the kidney, which in turn stimulates the bone marrow to produce more red cells. The baroreceptors are stretch receptors located in the walls of the aortic arch and the carotid sinus. Haemorrhage leads to a reduction in baroreceptor activity. Afferent information from these receptors travels via the IX cranial nerve to the vasomotor centre in the medulla. Reduced afferent activity leads to increased efferent output from the vasomotor centre via the sympathetic nervous system. The chemoreceptors are either central or peripheral. The former respond to pH and PaO_2 and are concerned with the control of respiration. The peripheral chemoreceptors, located in the aortic and carotid bodies, respond to hypoxaemia and hypoperfusion. Stimulation leads to increased sympathetic activity.

3.37   **Answers: A B C E**

The integrity of the baroreceptors and the autonomic nervous system can be tested by the Valsalva manoeuvre. The Valsalva manoeuvre is a forced expiration against a closed glottis. Initially this causes a transient rise in blood pressure as the rise in intrathoracic pressure expels a bolus of blood from the heart. The rise in intrathoracic pressure, however, reduces venous return and thus cardiac output and blood pressure drop. This is sensed by the baroreceptors which leads to increased sympathetic activity, vasoconstriction and tachycardia and a return of blood pressure towards normal. At the end of the Valsalva manoeuvre there is a transient rebound bradycardia and rise in blood pressure until the baroreceptors readjust. In patients with autonomic neuropathy, such as diabetics, there may be an abnormal response to the Valsalva manoeuvre.

3.38   **Answers: A D**

Potassium homeostasis is under the control of the hormone aldosterone. Potassium is excreted in very small amounts in health, it is filtered by the glomerulus and actively reabsorbed in the distal tubule. Postoperatively potassium excretion increases at least for the first few days.

3.39   **Answers: A D E**

There are three main clotting pathways: the intrinsic, extrinsic and common. The common pathway can be activated by either the extrinsic or intrinsic. The extrinsic pathway involves factor VII, whilst the intrinsic incorporates factors VIII, IX, XI and XII. The extrinsic path takes about 14 seconds, whilst the intrinsic is about twice as long. The common pathway is essentially the conversion of factor X to Xa. Factor Xa then converts prothrombin to thrombin, which in turn converts fibrinogen to fibrin. All the clotting factors are enzymes, many produced in the liver. Factors II, VII, IX and X are the vitamin K dependent factors.

3.40   **Answers: B D E**

Cerebrospinal fluid (CSF) is produced by the choroid plexus in the walls of the lateral ventricles at a rate of 0.4 ml/min. It is reabsorbed by the arachnoid villi. The volume of CSF is about 140 ml, about 10% of intracranial volume. The normal CSF pressure is 10–15 cm H_2O and varies with respiration and blood pressure.

3.41 **Answers: A B C D**

Both alcohol and mercury thermometers can be used to measure temperature. The Seebeck effect is employed in the thermocouple and resistance is used in both platinum resistance thermometers and thermistors.

3.42 **Answers: All false**

Boiling in water for 15 minutes at atmospheric pressure kills bacteria, but not spores. An autoclave pressure of 2–3 bar at 135°C for 3 minutes will kill all living organisms.

A 0.05% solution of chlorhexidine will sterilise an endotracheal tube in 30 minutes.

Ethylene oxide is effective against all organisms. At 55°C it takes about 2 hours, whilst at lower temperatures it takes up to 5 hours. In all cases, however, aeration takes a further 7 days.

3.43 **Answers: B D**

The Minimum Alveolar Concentration (MAC) is a concept first introduced by Eger and Merkel in 1963. MAC is the concentration of an anaesthetic agent that prevents the movement of 50% of the population to a standardised stimulus. It is measured at 1 atmosphere in fit, healthy male volunteers. It is an index of the potency of inhalational anaesthetic agents. The product of the oil/ gas coefficient and MAC is, for most agents, a constant. MAC of an agent is given as a volume %; for example the MAC of nitrous oxide is 105%. MAC is affected by a host of factors including age, other drugs, pyrexia and atmospheric pressure.

3.44 **Answer: B**

The body plethysmograph is used to measure airway resistance.

3.45 **Answers: All false**

Basal metabolic rate for an average adult male is about 20 kJ/m^2/hour. It is measured using a spirometer. Basal metabolic rate is higher in children and is increased by anxiety and in thyrotoxicosis. Not all patients with a goitre are thyrotoxic, indeed many are either hypothyroid or euthyroid. Basal metabolic rate is lower in the tropics.

3.46
Answers: C D

About 60% of an average 70 kg male is total body water; i.e. 42 litres. Of this, two-thirds is intracellular fluid and one-third is extracellular fluid. Two-thirds of extracellular fluid is interstitial and one-third is plasma volume. Plasma volume can be measured using Evans' blue or radioactively labelled albumin. The extracellular fluid volume can be measured with inulin. Inulin is also used to measure glomerular filtration rate (GFR). Creatinine is also often used to measure GFR. Para-amino hippuric acid is used to measure renal plasma flow.

3.47
Answers: A C E

Oxygen rotameters are variable orifice flowmeters. They consist of a bobbin in a cylinder and the scale along the side of the cylinder is non linear. Each rotameter is calibrated for the specific gas it will carry, although in theory it is possible to use nitrous oxide with an oxygen rotameter. Rotameters may be affected by back pressure.

3.48
Answers: A B C D E

Pressure is defined as force per unit area. Pressure can be expressed as Pascals (the SI unit of pressure), pounds per square inch (Imperial units) and bars.
A Pascal is equal to 1 kg/s^2, which in turn can be expressed as a Newton/m^2.

3.49
Answer: B

Oxygen and nitric oxide are attracted into a magnetic field; they are paramagnetic. This property is used in the paramagnetic analyser to measure the concentration of oxygen in a gas sample. These analysers are very accurate, sensitive and have a rapid response time.

3.50
Answers: A B C D E

The unit of electrical resistance is the Ohm. The Ohm is that resistance which will allow one ampere of current to flow under the influence of a potential of one volt. Ohm's law states that Resistance (R) = Potential (V)/Current (I). A rise in temperature increases the resistance of a wire resistor. Resistance rises as the tension or length of a wire increases.

3.51   **Answers: A C D**

Viscosity affects laminar flow according to the Hageni–Poiseuille formula. The viscosity of a liquid is inversely related to the temperature. With turbulent flow, density becomes the important factor. Heliox (oxygen/helium) is less dense than oxygen/nitrous oxide and is used to relieve inspiratory stridor where turbulent flow is a problem.

3.52   **Answer: C**

Surface tension is due to attraction between molecules in a liquid. It is measured in either newtons/metre or dynes/cm. It is independent of either temperature or viscosity. It leads to a mercury manometer under-reading.

3.53   **Answers: A D**

Boyle's law states that at constant temperature the volume of a fixed mass of gas varies inversely with the absolute pressure. A plot of P versus V is a rectangular hyperbole. One mole of any gas at standard temperature and pressure occupies 22.4 litres.

3.54   **Answers: A D**

Although widely used, mercury thermometers have a very slow response time, whereas platinum resistance thermometer probes have a very rapid response time. Thermistors can become unreliable if exposed to high temperatures.

3.55   **Answers: A B C D**

There are several ways of humidifying inspired gases including the nose! The artificial nose or heat and moisture exchanger (HME) is most commonly used in clinical practice. Other methods that have been employed include passage of gas through a cold or hot water bath or the use of nebulisers, some of which work by using the Bernoulli effect.

3.56　　　　　　　　　　　　　　　　　　　　**Answers: C D E**

The physical properties of nitrous oxide are:
Blood/gas solubility 0.47
MAC value of 105%
Filling ratio of 0.75
Critical temperature of 36.5°C
Critical pressure of 72.6 bar
Boiling point of –88°C

3.57　　　　　　　　　　　　　　　　　　　　　　**Answer: D**

To measure central venous pressure (CVP) a catheter is inserted via usually either the subclavian or internal jugular vein. When a reading is taken the patient should be lying flat and if connected to a ventilator, it should be taken at the end of expiration. The zero of the scale is the midaxillary line. The catheters tend to be long and narrow.

3.58　　　　　　　　　　　　　　　　　　　　　**Answers: A C**

Henry's law states that at a particular temperature the amount of a gas dissolved in a given liquid is directly proportional to the partial pressure of the gas in equilibrium with the liquid.

3.59　　　　　　　　　　　　　　　　　　　　　　**Answer: D**

Spirometry can be used to measure a number of lung volumes and lung capacities. It is the inspiratory reserve volume that can be measured; there is no functional in the title.

3.60　　　　　　　　　　　　　　　　　　　　**Answers: A B D E**

In circle systems the vaporiser may be located within the circle (VIC) or outside the circle (VOC). With a VIC, at low flows the vapour concentration will be higher than that dialled up. With a VOC the vapour concentration will be lower than that dialled up. It is thus important to monitor gas concentrations in a circle system.

3.61　　　　　　　　　　　　　　　　　　　　　　**Answer: B**

One atmosphere is equivalent to –1 bar, 101.3 kPa, 760 mmHg, 1000 cmH$_2$O, 14.7 Psi and 750 torr.

3.62   **Answer: C**

The intra-aortic balloon pump (IABP) is inserted via the femoral artery and positioned in the descending aorta, just distal to the left subclavian artery. Inflation is synchronised to the patients ECG. It is inflated with 50 ml of helium at the onset of diastole. This results in increased aortic diastolic pressure, improved coronary perfusion and improved myocardial oxygen delivery. Deflation occurs just prior to systole thus decreasing left ventricular afterload and left ventricular work.

3.63   **Answers: A D E**

Pacemakers may be affected by anaesthetic drugs, MRI scanners, shivering, diathermy and many other factors. Bipolar diathermy is safer than unipolar and MRI scanning is absolutely contraindicated in patients with a pacemaker. A demand pacemaker can readily be converted to a fixed rate pacemaker by placing a magnet over it.

3.64   **Answers: A B C D**

Entonox is the trade name for a 50:50 mixture of oxygen and nitrous oxide. It can be administered by registered midwives and is used for analgesia in labour. It is stored at a pressure of 137 bar and has a critical temperature of –7°C. Because of the Poynting effect the presence of oxygen reduces the critical temperature of nitrous oxide and at 137 bar the two gases dissolve in each other. Nitrous oxide inhibits the enzyme methionine synthetase and by this mechanism may, after prolonged exposure, cause megaloblastic anaemia.

3.65   **Answers: A B C D E**

The standard Tuohy needle is 16 G, has Lees lines every 1 cm and is 10 cm in length. At its tip is the Huber point and there may be Macintosh wings that can be attached to the needle. The bacterial filter has pores of 22 microns diameter. The epidural space may be located by the loss of resistance to air or saline technique or by the hanging drop method.

3.66   **Answers: B D**

In an exponential process after one time constant the value will have fallen to 37% of its original and after three time constants 95% of the process is complete.

3.67   **Answer: C**

Helium is stored as a gas at room temperature in brown cylinders at a pressure of 137 bar. It has a similar viscosity to oxygen but is far less dense. Its low density causes the voice changes seen when it is inhaled and makes it useful in upper airway obstruction such as stridor due to laryngeal obstruction. It is however of no value in treating bronchospasm. It does not support combustion nor is it narcotic at high pressure.

3.68   **Answers: A B D**

The Wright's respirometer is a turbine which measures gas volume, such as tidal or minute volume. It underreads at < 1 l/min and is affected by moisture which causes the pointer to stick. The pneumotachograph measures flow rate such as peak flow and is affected by gas viscosity.

3.69   **Answers: B C D E**

Peak flow is measured by the pneumotachograph. It has a normal diurnal variation and is reduced in an acute attack of asthma. The peak flow is usually used to monitor the response to therapy in an asthmatic. The measurement of peak flow is very dependent on effort.

3.70   **Answers: C E**

The Severinghaus electrode is used to measure the tension of carbon dioxide in blood; the $PaCO_2$. In fact, it is the concentration of hydrogen ions (the pH) that is actually measured but this is directly related to $PaCO_2$. The CO_2 in blood diffuses across a semi-permeable membrane and reacts with water to produce carbonic acid which then dissociates to hydrogen and bicarbonate ions. This reaction takes place at the pH sensitive glass electrode, which is bathed in bicarbonate ions. The pH is measured and from that the $PaCO_2$ is calculated.

3.71   **Answer: E**

Soda lime is used to absorb CO_2 in anaesthetic breathing systems. It contains approximately 90% calcium hydroxide. Sodium hydroxide (5%) and potassium hydroxide (1%) are present as catalysts for the reaction between soda lime and CO_2. An indicator dye is present to show when the soda lime is exhausted. The reaction is exothermic and produces heat. Soda lime is compatible with all the currently used volatile agents, although sevoflurane is degraded to compound A at high temperatures. Although nephrotoxic in rats there is no evidence that compound A is harmful to humans. Carboxyhaemoglobinaemia may occur when certain volatile agents react with dried out soda lime.

3.72   **Answers: A B C D E**

All of the options are potential complications of the siting of an arterial line.

3.73   **Answers: A B C D**

Thromboelastography is used to assess coagulation status. It is particularly useful in providing information on platelet function and fibrinolysis; neither of which are provided by the laboratory estimation of PT, APTT and platelet count. It takes, however, no longer to run than the laboratory tests. It is exquisitely sensitive to heparin, although any heparin effect can be blocked by adding heparinase reagent to the blood sample before running the TEG. The use of blood products such as FFP and platelets and the need for, for example, aprotinin or tranexamic acid can be ascertained from the TEG.

3.74   **Answers: A B C E**

The Transoesophageal Doppler probe employs high frequency sound waves. It can be used to assess cardiac output, segmental wall motion abnormalities and volaemic status. It is very sensitive to the presence of pulmonary emboli and can also be used to view heart valve anatomy.

3.75   **Answers: C E**

Microshock is the term used to describe the delivery of very small currents (100–150 microamps) directly to the myocardium, where they may cause ventricular fibrillation. Microshock requires the presence of a faulty intracardiac catheter (e.g. CVP line or pacemaker electrode) touching the wall of the heart along which current can flow.

Whilst 5% dextrose will not conduct current, saline certainly will. The severity of microshock is inversely related to current frequency so risk is greatest at low frequencies such as mains frequency.

3.76   **Answers: A C D E**

Halothane will absorb ultraviolet and infrared radiation and will cause a change in the elasticity of silicone rubber. Halothane concentration can also be determined by a refractometer. Halothane has a molecular weight of 197 Daltons: that of nitrous oxide is 44.

3.77   **Answers: A C D E**

In 1954, Mapleson devised a classification for the breathing systems in use. They were labelled A to E; the A is the Magill (or Lack coaxial version). It is the most efficient for spontaneous ventilation. The D system is the Bain and is the most efficient for controlled ventilation. The E is the Ayre's T piece and is the paediatric system used for children weighing less than 20 kg. This system was modified by Jackson-Rees who added an open ended bag; this became the F system.

3.78   **Answers: A B**

Nitrous oxide is stored in French blue cylinders made of molybdenum steel. The pressure at 20 °C is 54 bar; oxygen is stored at 137 bar. Because nitrous oxide is stored as a liquid it is present as a saturated vapour and the pressure in the cylinder only begins to fall once all the liquid has evaporated through use. The filling ratio is 0.67 and the critical temperature 36.5°C. The pin index number for cyclopropane was 3,6; that for nitrous oxide is 3,5.

3.79   Answers: A B D E

3.80   Answers: A E

Sellick's manoeuvre, or the application of cricoid pressure, is designed to prevent the passive regurgitation of acidic gastric contents. It requires the application of a force of 44 Newtons. It is performed by compressing the oesophagus between the cricoid cartilage and the vertebral body of C6; either as a one or two handed technique. It should not be applied if vomiting occurs as it may cause rupture of the oesophagus. Although it is sometimes used to aid visualisation of the cords it may have the opposite effect!

3.81   Answer: D

Pulse oximeters do not cause burns. They are inaccurate in the presence of both methaemoglobin and carboxyhaemoglobin but are unaffected by pigmented skin or the presence of fetal haemoglobin F.

3.82   Answers: A B

Disposable endotracheal tubes are implant tested on rabbits. The LMA may be re-used up to fifty times. The Fraser-Sweatman keyed filling devices are colour coded and the colour for isoflurane is purple.

3.83   Answer: D

The gas laws are as follows:
1) Boyle's law states that at constant temperature the volume of a gas is inversely proportional to the pressure.
2) Charles' law states that at constant pressure the volume of a gas is directly proportional to the temperature.
3) Gay-Lussac's law states that at constant volume the pressure of a gas is directly proportional to the temperature.

This leads to the combined (Universal) gas law: PV = kT, where k is a constant. Although not a gas law, Avogadro's hypothesis states that the gram molecular weight of a gas occupies 22.4 litres at standard temperature and pressure (STP).

3.84   **Answers: A D E**

The Hageni-Poiseuille formula relates to laminar flow of Newtonian fluids through a tube. The formula shows that flow is inversely related to viscosity; density is a factor only in turbulent, non laminar flow. Flow increases four fold for every doubling of diameter of the tube.

3.85   **Answers: A B D E**

Capnography, or the measurement of end-tidal CO_2, uses the principal of infrared absorption spectrophotometry. Infrared light is absorbed by any gas with two or more different atoms in the molecule, hence nitrous oxide will also absorb it. This is known as the Luft principle. The absorption spectra for infrared light for carbon dioxide and nitrous oxide are very close. The presence of a capnograph waveform reliably confirms the correct placement of an endotracheal tube

3.86   **Answers: A C**

Oxygen may be measured by fuel cell, mass spectrometer, paramagnetic analyser, chemically or polarographically. As oxygen has unpaired electrons it is attracted to a magnetic field (i.e. it is paramagnetic). Once in a magnetic field oxygen molecules become agitated, resulting in a change in pressure proportional to the oxygen concentration. This is detected by a transducer and converted into a displayed signal.

3.87   **Answers: A B**

The Mapleson E breathing system takes its name from its inventor Dr Philip Ayre who was a neuroanaesthetist in Newcastle, and designed it in 1937. It was later modified by Dr Jackson-Rees, an anaesthetist in Liverpool. He added an open ended bag to Ayre's T-piece. For efficient spontaneous respiration the fresh gas flow needs to be 2–3 times the patient's minute volume and, in addition, the volume of the corrugated tubing must exceed the patient's tidal volume. It should be used in children of 20 kg or less. Although scavenging from the system is possible, it is not particularly easy.

3.88   **Answers: A B C D E**

The critical temperature is the temperature above which a gas cannot be liquefied by pressure.

3.89   **Answers: A B C**

The pin-index system was designed to prevent the wrong gas cylinder being attached to an anaesthetic machine. One or more pins project from the yoke and these fit into holes on the cylinder. The configuration of the pins is specific to each gas.

Oxygen is 2,5
Cyclopropane 3,6
Nitrous oxide 3,5
Helium no pin
Entonox a single pin.

3.90   **Answers: A B C E**

Nitrous oxide was discovered by Joseph Priestley in 1772 and its anaesthetic properties were first suggested in 1799 by another Englishman, Sir Humphrey Davy. It was first used as an anaesthetic in 1844; just 21 months before the first use of ether. It is a sweet smelling, non-irritant gas which though not explosive will support combustion. It has a boiling point of –88°C, a critical temperature of 36.5 and a critical pressure of 72.6 bar. Its MAC value is 105%. It is supplied from pipelines at a pressure of 4 bar or from cylinders, stored at a pressure of 54 bar.

STATION 3.1

Answers and explanations

(a) The likely diagnosis is meningococcal septicaemia.

(b) The purpuric rash that accompanies the illness means that there is abnormal clotting and probably disseminated intravascular coagulation (DIC). Urgent blood cultures should be sent for confirmation of the diagnosis and a full blood count and clotting screen to confirm and quantify the clotting problem.

(c) The management involves the administration of intravenous antibiotics without waiting for microbiological confirmation of the diagnosis. Usually benzylpenicillin is the antibiotic of choice, but a third line cephalosporin is also a reasonable alternative. To treat the coagulopathy platelets, fresh frozen plasma (FFP) and cryoprecipitate may be needed. Usually intravenous fluids and inotropic support are required; there may be a need to intubate and ventilate.

STATION 3.2

Answers and explanations

(a) This lady has acute liver failure secondary to an overdose of paracetamol.

(b) Normally a toxic intermediate produced by the metabolism of paracetamol is detoxified by conjugation with glutathione, produced in the liver. In overdose, however, the glutathione is exhausted leaving the toxic intermediate free to wreak havoc on the hepatocytes. The liver is important in synthesising certain proteins including many of the clotting factors. Thus in liver failure a coagulopathy develops. Another function of the liver is the regulation of carbohydrate metabolism and gluconeogenesis. Hypoglycaemia frequently accompanies acute hepatic failure and, unless corrected may lead to coma.

(c) She should be referred to a specialist liver unit for further management.

(d) This lady requires immediate intravenous glucose, correction of her coagulopathy and intravenous acetylcysteine to replenish glutathione stores.

STATION 3.3

Answers and explanations

(a) This is 2,6-di-isopropylphenol.
It is presented commercially as an aqueous emulsion containing glycerol, purified egg phosphatide and soya bean oil.

(b) The main side-effects are:
Pain on injection; this is reduced by adding lignocaine to the propofol
Hypotension, due to peripheral vasodilatation
Respiratory depression

STATION 3.4

Answers and explanations

The arterial and venous blood samples show very marked hyperglycaemia and a metabolic acidosis. In addition there is a neutrophil leucocytosis and an elevated urea and creatinine.

(a) Diabetic ketoacidosis, assuming that there are the confirmatory ketones in the urine.

(b) This patient should be managed with insulin and intravenous fluids.

(c) The likely trigger is an infection, hence the neutrophil leucocytosis. The likely sources of infection are the urinary tract and the lungs. Appropriate antibiotics will be needed to treat the underlying infection.

(d) Diabetic ketoacidosis is more likely in type 1 or insulin dependent diabetics, whilst type 2 diabetics, who are usually controlled with either diet or oral hypoglycaemic drugs, tend to present in hyperosmolar, non-ketotic coma.

STATION 3.5

Answers and explanations

(a) The ECG shows the typical changes associated with the Wolff–Parkinson–White syndrome; a short PR interval, a delta wave and a widened QRS complex.

(b) Patients with this condition are at danger of developing tachyarrhythmias such as supraventricular tachycardia and atrial fibrillation.

(c) Pre-operatively it is necessary to have these patients seen by a cardiologist, who may start appropriate medication to prevent the occurrence of the aforementioned arrhythmias.

STATION 3.6

Answers and explanations

The assessment consists of taking a history, performing a physical examination and looking at the results of relevant investigations.

When taking the history one would enquire about the frequency and severity of angina; what medications the man takes and whether he has ever suffered a full blown myocardial infarction, and if so, when. One would enquire about exercise tolerance and any symptoms suggestive of coexistent cardiac failure such as orthopnoea, ankle swelling and paroxysmal nocturnal dyspnoea.

In the physical examination one would listen for murmurs, signs of heart failure, look for an elevated jugular venous pressure, assess the rate, quality and rhythm of the arterial pulse and feel for the apex beat.

Relevant investigations would include a 12 lead ECG and chest X-ray. If indicated, further tests might include a stress test ECG, coronary angiography and an echocardiogram to assess overall cardiac function and ejection fraction.

STATION 3.7

Answers and explanations

(a) This is a vial of sodium nitroprusside.
(b) It should be stored in the dark.
(c) It is degraded by light.
(d) It is used to reduce blood pressure for hypotensive anaesthesia.
(e) It is reconstituted in 5% dextrose and should be used within 24 hours of preparation.
(f) It should be protected from light during use.
(g) The dosage is 0.1–5 µg/kg/min i.v.
(h) The maximum dose is 8 µg/kg/min.
(i) The danger of prolonged use is cyanide toxicity.
(j) This presents as a marked metabolic acidosis and is treated with dicobalt edetate.

STATION 3.8

Answers

(a) True   **(b) False**   **(c) True**   **(d) True**
The ECG shows an acute inferoposterior MI with lateral ischaemia. There is evidence of first degree heart block and such ischaemia predisposes to various degrees of atrioventricular nodal block. The patient should be treated with aspirin and, if no contraindications, thrombolysis.

STATION 3.9

Answers and explanations

1.
(a) The lady is clearly thyrotoxic. She has exophthalmos and appears to have a large thyroid goitre too. This would suggest she is suffering from Graves' disease.

(b) Systemic corticosteroids or local radiotherapy may be required to treat the eye condition, which may not regress once she is rendered euthyroid. Biochemical testing in this lady would reveal an elevated T4 and a low TSH. Before surgery she should be treated with an antithyroid drug such as carbimazole.

(c) Clinical examination is likely to reveal that she is in atrial fibrillation or at least a sinus tachycardia; she may require treatment with a beta blocker; there may be a thyroid bruit and there is usually hyperreflexia.

2.
(a) This man is suffering from hypothyroidism and has a very large thyroid goitre.
Biochemistry reveals a low T4 and elevated TSH.

(b) Clinical signs include a toad like facies, bradycardia, slow relaxing reflexes and a goitre.

(c) With such a large goitre one might anticipate a difficult intubation and a gaseous induction or awake fibreoptic intubation should therefore be considered.

(d) Post-operative problems include damage to the recurrent laryngeal nerves, tracheal collapse from tracheomalacia and haemorrhage; all of these may lead to post-operative airway obstruction.

STATION 3.10

Answers and explanations

(a) The X-ray of the femur shows the typical bowing and increased bone density of Paget's disease.

(b) Paget's disease is caused by increased bone turnover and is associated with fractures and, rarely, with sarcoma formation in affected bones. It may lead to a high output cardiac failure which is its main relevance to anaesthesia.

STATION 3.11

Answers and explanations

(a) Figure 3.11 shows clubbing of the fingers.

(b) This clinical sign is associated with a wide range of clinical conditions, in particular suppurative lung disease may lead to clubbing. Pulmonary tuberculosis, cystic fibrosis, bronchial carcinoma and bronchiectasis are all causes. Patients with lung disease may require intensive physiotherapy pre- and post-operatively and avoidance of drugs that cause respiratory depression.

(c) Cyanotic congenital heart disease is another cause of clubbing and this would clearly affect the anaesthetic given. Intra-abdominal pathology is associated with clubbing such as ulcerative colitis, Crohn's and liver cirrhosis. A cirrhotic patient is likely to have abnormal clotting, hyponatraemia and hypoalbuminaemia which have implications for anaesthesia.

STATION 3.12

Answers and explanations

(a) ECT has effects on the central nervous system (CNS) and the cardiovascular system (CVS). CNS effects: increased cerebral metabolic rate, intracranial pressure and blood flow. CVS effects: initially increased parasympathetic activity with bradycardia and hypotension which may even result in asystole. This is followed by increased sympathetic activity with hypertension and tachycardia, lasting about 10 minutes. Cardiac output and myocardial oxygen consumption are increased, cardiac ischaemia and even myocardial infarction may be precipitated. Atrial and ventricular arrhythmias can occur.

(b) Myocardial infarction within 3 months and cerebrovascular accident within 3 months are contraindications to ECT. Relative contraindications include the presence of ischaemic heart disease or other cardiac pathology.

STATION 3.13

Answer and explanation

A Biers block or intravenous regional anaesthesia (IVRA) is a technique used to anaesthetise the lower part of the arm (or leg). The patient should have the technique fully explained to her.
The usual monitoring must be in place and emergency drugs and equipment must be to hand.
An intravenous cannula is sited in both arms; the one on the affected side to administer local anaesthesia.
Over the affected arm a double cuff is placed and the proximal one is inflated to 100 mm Hg above systolic.
0.5% Prilocaine is injected via the cannula in the affected arm at a dose of 3 mg/kg. Whilst injecting, the patient is asked about any symptoms suggestive of toxicity, such as peri-oral paraesthesiae. Once the injection is finished the distal cuff is inflated and after that the proximal is deflated to minimise tourniquet pain.
At the end of the operation, as long as at least 25 mins has elapsed since injection of prilocaine, the distal cuff is deflated.

STATION 3.14

Answers and explanations

(a) Soda lime is a compound used in anaesthetic breathing systems to absorb carbon dioxide and allow recycling of anaesthetic gases. Soda lime is used particularly in circle systems.

Soda lime consists of
Sodium hydroxide	5%
Calcium hydroxide	80%
Potassium hydroxide	1%
Water	14%

The potassium hydroxide is a catalyst for the reaction between soda lime and carbon dioxide:

$$2NaOH + CO_2 \rightarrow Na_2CO_3 + H_2O, \text{ then}$$
$$Na_2CO_3 + Ca(OH)_2 \rightarrow CaCO_3 + 2NaOH$$

The reaction is exothermic and produces heat, up to 60°C in the centre of a soda lime canister.

(b) One of the advantages of circle systems is that the heat and water generated keeps the patient warm and prevents drying up of secretions and sputum in the tracheobronchial tree. The soda lime contains an indicator dye to show when it is exhausted. Using circle systems is economical as the gases are recycled. Circle systems are said to be environmentally friendly as most anaesthetic agents are greenhouse gases.

STATION 3.15

Answer

The Association of Anaesthetists of Great Britain and Ireland have published guidelines on checking the anaesthetic machine; these are printed below. They should be studied and remembered so that the perfect answer is available for when you are asked this question!

GUIDELINES ON CHECKING THE ANAESTHETIC MACHINE

The following checks should be carried out at the beginning of each operating theatre session. **These checks are the responsibility of the anaesthetist and must not be delegated to other personnel.** In the event of a change of anaesthetist during an operating session the checked status of the anaesthetic machine must be agreed.

Before using any anaesthetic apparatus, ventilator, breathing system or monitor, it is essential to be fully familiar with it. This familiarisation process, which may entail study of the instruction manual, is particularly important when faced with new equipment and should be regarded as an essential part of the safety check. Similarly, a thorough understanding must be gained of any equipment assembled in an unfamiliar configuration.

A   ANAESTHETIC MACHINE

Check that the anaesthetic machine and relevant ancillary equipment are connected to the mains electrical supply (where appropriate) and switched. Careful note should be taken of any information or labelling on the anaesthetic machine which might refer to its current status.

B   OXYGEN ANALYSER

1. The oxygen analyser should be placed where it can monitor the composition of the gases leaving the common gas outlet.
2. The analyser should be switched on, checked and calibrated according to the manufacturer's instructions.

C   MEDICAL GAS SUPPLIES

1. Identify and take note of the gases which are being supplied by pipeline, confirming with a 'tug test' that each pipeline is correctly inserted into the appropriate gas supply.
2. Check that the anaesthetic apparatus is connected to a supply of oxygen and that an adequate reserve supply of oxygen is available from a spare cylinder.

3. Check that adequate supplies of any other gases intended for use are available and connected as appropriate. All cylinders should be securely seated and turned OFF after checking their contents.
    Carbon dioxide cylinders should not normally be present on the anaesthetic machine. A blanking plug should be fitted to any empty cylinder yoke.

4. All pressure gauges for pipelines connected to the anaesthetic machine should indicate 400 kPa.

5. Check the operation of flowmeters, ensuring that each control valve operates smoothly and that the bobbin moves freely throughout its range without sticking. With only the oxygen flow control valve open and a flow of approximately 5 litres per minute, check that the oxygen analyser display approaches 100%. Turn off all flow control valves.

6. Operate the emergency oxygen bypass control and ensure that flow occurs without significant decrease in the pipeline supply pressure. Confirm that the oxygen analyser display approaches 100% during this test. Ensure that the emergency oxygen bypass control ceases to operate when released.

D   VAPORISERS

1. Check that the vaporiser(s) for the required volatile agent(s) are fitted correctly to the anaesthetic machine, that any back bar locking mechanism is fully engaged and that the control knobs rotate fully through the full range(s). Ensure that the vaporiser is not tilted. Turn off the vaporisers.

2. Check that the vaporiser(s) are adequately filled and that the filling port is tightly closed.

3. (i)   Set a flow of oxygen of 5 litres/min and, with the vaporiser turned off, temporarily occlude the common gas outlet. There should be no leak from any of the vaporiser fitments and the flowmeter bobbin should dip.
    (ii) Turn each vaporiser on in turn and repeat this test. There should be no leak of liquid from the filling port. After this test, ensure that the vaporisers and flowmeters are turned off.
    (iii) Should it be necessary to change a vaporiser at any stage, it is essential to repeat the leak test. Failure to do so is one of the commonest causes of critical incidents.
    (iv) Removal of a vaporiser from a machine in order to refill it is not considered necessary.

E   BREATHING SYSTEM

1. Check all breathing systems which are to be employed. They should be visually inspected for correct configuration and assembly. All connections within the system and to the anaesthetic machine should be secured by 'push and twist'. Ensure that there are no leaks or obstructions in the reservoir bags or breathing system. A pressure leak test should be performed on the breathing system by occluding the patient end and compressing the

reservoir bag. Each breathing system poses separate problems. Each should be checked as appropriate and in particular it is necessary to perform an occlusion test on the inner tube of the Bain-type coaxial system, to ensure that it is correctly attached.

2.   Check that the adjustable pressure limiting 'expiratory' valve can be fully opened and closed.
3.   The correct operation of the unidirectional valves in a circle system should be carefully checked.
4.   If it is intended to use very low fresh gas flows in a circle breathing system, there must be a means to analyse the oxygen concentration in the inspiratory limb. End tidal CO_2 and agent concentration must also be monitored in this situation.

F   VENTILATOR

1.   Check that the ventilator is configured correctly for its intended use. Ensure that the ventilator tubing is securely attached. Set the controls for use and ensure that adequate pressure is generated during the inspiratory phase.
2.   Check that a disconnect alarm is present and functions correctly.
3.   Check that the pressure relief valve functions correctly at the set pressure.
4.   Ensure that there is an alternative means to ventilate the patient's lungs in the event of ventilator malfunction.

G   SCAVENGING

The anaesthetic gas scavenging system should be switched on and functioning. Ensure that the tubing is attached to the appropriate expiratory port of the breathing system or ventilator.

H   ANCILLARY EQUIPMENT

1.   All ancillary equipment which may be needed should be present, such as laryngoscopes, intubation aids (intubation forceps, bougies), etc. Ensure that all sizes of face masks, airways, tracheal tubes and connectors are available.
2.   Check that all laryngoscopes are working.
3.   The suction apparatus must be functioning and all connections should be secure; test for the rapid development of an adequate negative pressure.
4.   Check that the patient trolley, bed or operating table can be rapidly tilted head-down.

I   MONITORING

1.   Ensure that the appropriate monitoring equipment is present, switched on and calibrated.
2.   Set all necessary alarm limits, as appropriate.

The above information has been reproduced by kind permission of the Association of Anaesthetists of Great Britain and Ireland.

STATION 3.16

Answer and explanation

The patient should be told that it is perfectly possible to do the operation without any pain using any of the aforementioned techniques. Whilst a spinal is a one off technique, an epidural or CSE has the advantage of longevity of analgesia. Thus with an epidural or CSE the length of operation is not a limiting factor and, in addition, the epidural catheter can be used to provide post-operative pain relief. In terms of performing the blocks the techniques are almost identical. An i.v. drip should be set up and the patient monitored as usual.

Viva 3a

PHARMACOLOGY
Anti-emetics

What neurotransmitters are involved in nausea and vomiting? Where would we encounter them?
Neurotransmitters involved in nausea and vomiting can be thought of as central or peripheral. Centrally (inside the blood-brain barrier) is the vomiting centre which has muscarinic acetylcholine receptors and histamine receptors. The chemoreceptor trigger zone (which lies outside the blood-brain barrier) has dopamine (D2) and 5-HT3 receptors. Peripherally in the stomach there are dopamine and 5-HT3 receptors.

Classify anti-emetics by their mechanism of action. Where are their main sites of action?
Dopamine antagonists: metoclopramide, prochlorperazine, droperidol, domperidone
Antihistamines: promethazine, cyclizine
Anticholinergics: hyoscine
5-HT3 antagonists: ondansetron, granisetron, (? Metoclopramide in high doses)
Corticosteroids: dexamethasone
Cannabinoid: nabilone

How can we administer anti-emetics?
Anti-emetics can be given orally, intravenously, intramuscularly, rectally or transdermally.

Do you know of any drugs that can be administered transdermally?
Fentanyl, glyceryl trinitrate, amethocaine (Ametop), prilocaine and lignocaine (EMLA), hormone replacement therapy.

PHYSIOLOGY
Gastric motility

What factors control gastric emptying?
Gastric emptying is controlled by both neural and hormonal mechanisms.

Neural (immediate response)
- Parasympathetic (vagal): promotes gastric emptying
- Sympathetic: inhibits gastric emptying
- Intrinsic myenteric plexus

Hormonal (slower, sustained response)
- Gastrin: promotes gastric emptying
- Secretin, cholecystokinin (CCK), **glucose**-dependent **insulin**-releasing **peptide** (GIP): inhibit gastric emptying

Gastric factors increasing gastric emptying
- Increase gastric motility and relax pyloric sphincter
- Gastric distension

Neural: increased gastric motility and relaxation of pyloric sphincter
Hormonal: gastrin secretion in response to certain foods especially proteins
Direct: effect on gastric smooth muscle excitability
- Fluidity of gastric contents: increased fluidity stimulates gastric emptying
- Type of food: carbohydrates spend the least time in the stomach, then proteins and lastly fat

Duodenal factors inhibiting gastric emptying
- Decrease gastric motility and cause pyloric sphincter contraction
- Enterogastric reflex (intrinsic nerve plexuses and autonomic nervous system)
- Hormonal: CCK, secretin, GIP release
- Fat
- Acidity
- Hypertonicity: neural or hormonal response; decreased gastric emptying
- Distension
- Irritation

Higher centres
- Sight, smell, thought of food: parasympathetics – increased gastric emptying
- Pain, fear: sympathetics - decreased gastric emptying

What would therefore promote gastric stasis?
Pathophysiological
- Pain, trauma, shock, anxiety
- Cold stress
- Labour
- Depression

Pathological
- Gastrointestinal obstruction: pyloric stenosis, duodenal obstruction
- Pseudo-obstruction: collagen diseases, amyloidosis
- Acute abdomen: peritonitis, pancreatitis, splenic rupture, retroperitoneal haematoma
- Acute gastroparesis: gastro-enteritis, ketoacidosis, electrolyte imbalance, hyperglycaemia, acute renal failure
- Diabetic autonomic neuropathy
- Hypothyroidism

Pharmacological
- Opioids
- Anticholinergics: atropine, phenothiazines, tricyclic anti-depressants
- Sympathomimetics: isoprenaline, salbutamol, adrenaline
- Dopamine
- Alcohol
- Aluminium, magnesium

Describe the vomiting act
- Reverse peristalsis starting from as distal as the ileum
- Relaxation of pyloric sphincter and stomach to allow small intestinal contents to enter the stomach
- Overdistension of the duodenum and stomach – initiates the vomiting act
- Deep breath held and glottis closes to prevent entry of vomitus into lungs
- Soft palate raised to close nasopharynx
- Pyloric sphincter contracts to prevent flow
- Diaphragm contracts downwards and at the same time abdominal and thoracic muscles contract, compressing the stomach and increasing intragastric pressure
- Oesophageal sphincters relax
- Expulsion of the gastric contents

Viva 3b

CLINICAL

What is your initial management?
The management of status epilepticus comprises controlling the seizures, securing the airway and then investigating the cause of the seizures.

Intravenous access must be secured and an anticonvulsant such as Diazemuls (5–20 mg) should be given intravenously to terminate the seizures.

The airway should be maintained and oxygen given.

If seizures persist and the airway is compromised the patient should be intubated.

Thiopentone is a useful agent both to induce sleep prior to intubation and as an anticonvulsant.

Monitoring including ECG, pulse oximetry and non-invasive blood pressure should be instituted.

If seizures continue despite the above, then a phenytoin infusion can be started, following a loading dose and bearing in mind that hypotension and dysrhythmias are common with this drug.

Investigations include a BM stix and blood glucose estimation to exclude hypoglycaemia.

Electrolytes including calcium to exclude hyponatraemia or hypocalcaemia.

Urea and creatinine and a full toxicology screen should be requested.

Alcohol intoxication and withdrawal can both cause seizures as can drugs such as amphetamines, Ecstasy, tricyclic antidepressants and theophyllines.

In a known epileptic, anticonvulsant levels should be measured to check that the fits are not due to subtherapeutic levels of anticonvulsants.

A CT or MRI scan of the brain should be carried out in anyone presenting in this way for the first time with no obvious cause to exclude an intracerebral lesion such as a tumour.

What are the common causes of seizures?
25% are idiopathic.
The other 75% may be due to a brain lesion (tumour, abscess or haemorrhage), alcohol withdrawal, drug intoxication or metabolic cause.

PHYSICS
Defibrillators

What is a defibrillator? How does it work?
A defibrillator is a device used to deliver an electric shock to the heart which causes synchronous depolarisation of most or all of the heart muscle cells to try to convert an abnormal rhythm (ventricular fibrillation, ventricular tachycardia, atrial fibrillation or flutter) to a normal rhythm. Basically it consists of a power source capable of providing direct current (usually a rechargeable battery) and a capacitor which stores electrical charge and which may subsequently be discharged through external (applied to chest wall) or internal (direct contact with the heart) defibrillator paddles or adhesive electrodes. Direct current is used as it has been shown to be more effective, causes less myocardial damage and is less arrhythmogenic than alternating current.

What types of defibrillators are generally available? What are their advantages and disadvantages?
Manual defibrillators: where the operator interprets the rhythm and decides on whether defibrillation is necessary. The operator has to set the energy required and apply the paddles to electrodes on the chest. They require training and skill to operate.
Automated external defibrillators: analyse the rhythm and give instructions on a screen or by voice. The operator has to recognise cardiac arrest and stick the electrodes on the chest. The electrodes monitor the heart and give the defibrillatory shock. These defibrillators even charge themselves to the appropriate energy level. They generally have a manual override. These machines have a very high specificity for recognising shockable rhythms (~90%). Useful for those not fully trained in ECG interpretation. However they may mistake very fine ventricular fibrillation for asystole.
Automated implantable cardiac defibrillators: a miniaturised implanted defibrillator which senses and shocks (10–20 J) ventricular fibrillation and ventricular tachycardia via transvenous leads in patients especially at risk. It contains its own power source.

Shock advisory defibrillators: halfway between manual and automatic defibrillators. They analyse the heart rhythm and instruct the operator to charge the defibrillator to the appropriate energy level if a shock is required and deliver the shock to the patient.

Biphasic defibrillators: here the polarity of the current is reversed part of the way through delivery of the shock. This lowers the defibrillation threshold and allows less energy to be delivered for successful defibrillations so that these machines are safer, smaller and more portable as they contain smaller capacitors. They also have a longer refractory period which helps to block fibrillating wave-fronts.

Why are our first two shocks only 200 Joules in the VF/VT guidelines?

An initial 200 J shock has been shown to result in successful defibrillation in most remediable situations and causes minimal myocardial damage (an excessive amount of energy may damage the heart and other tissues or lead to unresponsive arrhythmias). Thoracic impedance is decreased by the first shock and so a second shock at the same energy setting will deliver greater energy to the heart.

MCQ REVISION INDEX

The number against each item refers to the examination and question number.